SUCCESSFUL HOME BIRTH AND MIDWIFERY

Successful Home Birth and Midwifery

The Dutch Model

Edited by
Eva Abraham-Van der Mark

Foreword by Brigitte Jordan

BERGIN & GARVEY
Westport, Connecticut • London

Library of Congress Cataloging-in-Publication Data

Successful home birth and midwifery : the Dutch model /
  edited by Eva Abraham-Van der Mark ; foreword by Brigitte Jordan.
    p. cm.
  Includes bibliographical references and index.
  ISBN 0-89789-295-X (alk. paper)
    1. Maternal health services—Netherlands. 2. Childbirth at home—
Netherlands. 3. Midwives—Netherlands. I. Abraham-Van der Mark,
Eva.
  RG964.N4S83 1993
  618.2'009492—dc20   92–42901

British Library Cataloguing in Publication Data is available.

Library of Congress Catalog Card Number: 92–42901
ISBN: 0-89789-295-X

First published in 1993

Bergin & Garvey, 88 Post Road West, Westport, CT 06881
An imprint of Greenwood Publishing Group, Inc.

Printed in the United States of America

The paper used in this book complies with the
Permanent Paper Standard issued by the National
Information Standards Organization (Z39.48–1984).

10 9 8 7 6 5 4 3 2 1

NWST
IAEA 6102

To the memory of
Astrid Limburg, midwife
October 13, 1939–February 8, 1993

Contents

Foreword

For those of us who have been involved in attempts to come to an understanding of the birth process that goes beyond the medical model, the Dutch way of birth has always been an inspiration. In most of the industrialized Western world, progress in obstetrics has been measured in increasing levels of intervention, in escalating technologization, and in the almost complete removal of the birth process from the domain of the woman and the family into the realm of technocratic specialists. To imagine that there exists an industrialized country with all the resources of modern medicine, of pharmacology, technology, and surgery, whose professionals subscribe to a scientific view of the world and whose citizens have a standard of living that easily puts at their disposal all the resources of technologized obstetrics, that there is such a country and that its women and care providers actively espouse a noninterventionist stance in childbirth—that has always been one of the great puzzles, paradoxes, and revelations in our field.

The book you are about to read will go far in explaining this most anomalous phenomenon. It traces the development of Dutch obstetrics and midwifery to its historical roots in the Middle Ages and outlines its development in the recent past. Though Dutch midwives suffered a decrease in status when they were stripped of the power to baptize, what is striking is that their legally defined sphere of competence and their autonomy from the medical profession have actually increased throughout the years, most recently (in 1987) with the power to decide what constitutes normal and abnormal birth.

This course of development contrasts starkly with what happened in the United States, where midwifery as an independent profession was wiped out by the middle of this century, surviving only for some time in the granny mid-wives of the rural South. In the last few years, however, we have seen a revi-val of midwifery in a variety of forms in America, from Certified Nurse Midwives (many of whom work in the large inner-city hospitals that serve the poor) to community-based empirical midwives who carry on the almost ex-tinct tradition of responsible home birth. Though outcome evaluations are dif-ficult to come by and not easily judged, it appears that planned, midwife-attended home birth is a safe alternative to hospital delivery in the United States as well.

Worldwide, however, the most disturbing trend is that midwife-attended home birth and midwife-attended clinic birth have been undermined by the claims and the prestige of high-technology medicine, as carried out by obstet-ric specialists. Typically, this has taken the form of a political struggle that pitched a male-dominated profession against only loosely organized midwife associations, with the result that in some countries midwifery has been elimi-nated for all practical purposes; in others, it has been co-opted so that mid-wives now perform the services and functions defined as preparatory and auxiliary, while technical procedures and the actual delivery are reserved for the physician. The midwife has thus become an assistant to the physician, not the woman.

This did not happen in the Netherlands. There was always a good national consensus among Dutch people, shared by the majority of obstetricians, that normal birth should take place at home, attended by midwives, while patho-logical deliveries should take place in hospitals, attended by obstetricians. What the Dutch have that is lacking in almost all other maternity care sys-tems is, first, an effective mechanism that allows them to separate out fore-seeably pathological deliveries from normal births, and second, universal maternity services that include comprehensive prenatal care and practical postpartum assistance in the home where necessary. These features deserve widespread discussion and consideration.

In the Third World, indigenous obstetric systems are increasingly over-whelmed by the prestigious, high-technology cosmopolitan obstetric model of the United States and most European countries. Yet it is also clear that much of the new technology does not contribute to better outcomes for mothers and babies, but rather is the source of medically generated injuries and prob-lems. In particular where the infrastructure for carrying out high-technology procedures is lacking, as it is in almost all developing countries, emphasis on technology leads only to further damage. It also leads to a principled devalua-tion of the expertise and wisdom inherent in indigenous ethno-obstetric sys-tems and of the empirical skills of native midwives who, in fact, have much to teach us. I have advocated for years that the Dutch example of maternity care is much more appropriate for developing countries than the Euro-American, technocratic, physician-dominated model.

I hope that this book will be read not only by those already convinced of the value of family centered, home-oriented, low-intervention pregnancy care and childbirth, but also by some of the practitioners who rely on the control provided by technology for the "management" of the process. Keeping in mind that the Dutch have one of the very best records in pregnancy outcome statistics, the "midwifery model of birth," described in its various forms in this book, might give those who are unfamiliar with its record food for thought, and for a renewed and active questioning of the practices whose benefits we often take for granted.

It is always of tremendous value to be able to step outside one's own cherished assumptions and ingrained practices to see that the world could be constructed otherwise and that that might not be disastrous. This book lays out an alternate model, an alternate vision, indeed an alternate reality of pregnancy and birth that puts those of other parts of the world into perspective. Let it provide inspiration for rethinking what good obstetric care could be like around the world.

Acknowledgments

I am extremely grateful to the Netherlands Organization of Midwives (NOV) and the Catharina Schrader Foundation for their financial support, which made it possible to have our English made into proper American. The Catharina Schrader Foundation, named for the famous Dutch midwife who left us her fascinating diary, is dedicated to promoting wider knowledge of the midwifery profession and encouraging scholarly research on midwifery.

Midwife Annemiek Cuppen read all chapters of the manuscript and provided valuable information and criticism. Midwife Astrid Limburg taught me about midwifery and much more than that, she showed me what a great profession it is. It is terribly sad that I will not have the opportunity to keep my promise of bringing her a copy of the book. Astrid was born at home in 1939 and died at home in February 1993. She has been a great source of inspiration for all those who care about home birth and midwifery, in the Netherlands and abroad. She lectured in many countries, especially in the United States and Canada. Through her "Office of Foreign Affairs," people all over the world were sent information and answers to their questions, streams of visitors were received, and many of them were introduced to the Dutch model in practice.

I owe a particular debt to Sonja Damstra-Wijmenga who was always ready to help, encourage and provide information. Her research, carried out in Groningen, is convincing proof of the safety of home birth.

Phyllis Mitzman made our English texts into American English. Marlene Dumas and Paul Andriesse have been extremely generous in allowing me to choose from their art, and Astrid Limburg, Mrs. E. J. Schaepman-Van Geuns,

Floor van Gelder, and the Museum Boymans-van Beuningen provided photographs.

Kathryn Fletcher stimulated this project when she, among others, asked me for a list of books in English on Dutch home birth and midwifery. I then realized that such books did not exist.

I regret that Fransje Van der Waals was not able to continue working with me on this book and I thank her for what she has done. Rineke Van Daalen has often listened to my lamentations and helped to solve various problems.

Finally, I want to thank the man who has made an enormous contribution to the Dutch model as it is described in this book: Professor G. J. Kloosterman. A couple of times friends asked me how I was getting on with "the Kloostermanbook." It is in a sense his book, and I hope that he will be satisfied with its contents.

SUCCESSFUL HOME BIRTH AND MIDWIFERY

1

Introduction to the Dutch System of Home Birth and Midwifery

Eva Abraham-Van der Mark

The history of childbirth in the Netherlands and the unbroken importance of home delivery in Dutch society are unique. Compared to other Western industrialized countries, the Netherlands has a very high percentage of home births. One-third of all babies are born at home. The practice of home birth is associated with low maternal and infant mortality. Medical interventions are minimal. Along with high regard for home delivery are the respect and status accorded to midwives, who are autonomous medical practitioners.

GIVING BIRTH: A NORMAL PHYSIOLOGICAL PROCESS

In 1991 the percentage of home births in the Netherlands was 33.4 against less than 4 percent in other Western industrialized countries.[1] Home birth is based on the conception of pregnancy and delivery as natural physiological processes. The basic assumption is that it is normal for a woman's body to do the work of labor and delivery. Moreover, emphasis is placed on the importance of a relaxed and familiar setting, preferably the home. When a woman gives birth at home, the doctor or midwife assisting is her guest; the woman must remain in control of her environment and be the center. An unfamiliar setting, such as a hospital, diminishes the woman's autonomy and self-confidence. She becomes a patient and is required to adjust to the rules of the institution. In a hospital, the medical personnel are in control, and the easy availability of drugs and medical technology promote unnecessary intervention. In a clinical setting, there exists a strong inclination towards taking action and "getting things done."[2] Home birth, on the other hand, assumes

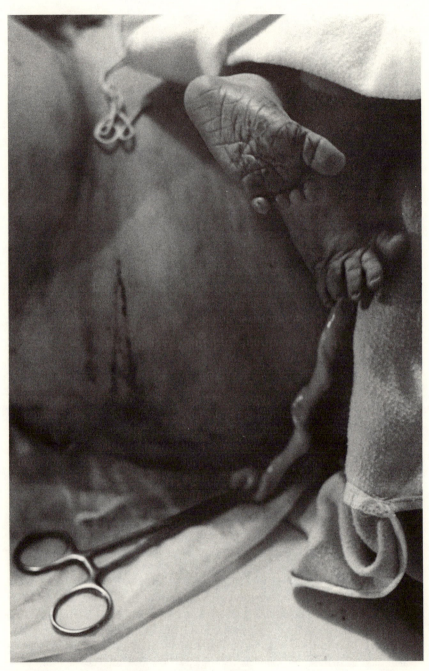

"Bonding," 1992. Copyright © by Paul Andriesse.

that giving birth is normal: The natural method is to be preferred over drugs. Medical intervention and the use of anesthesia are reserved for cases considered to be pathological. The present system is an accommodation between high and low obstetric technology. As a rule, the former is employed by obstetricians for problematic births, and the latter by midwives for those that are normal. Rates of medical interventions are considerably lower than in other countries (Treffers in this volume), which is related to expectative obstetrics and the position of midwives who are considered the guardians of normal birth without intervention (chapters by Marland and Abraham in this volume). Expectative obstetrics values patience in the belief that in a normal birth, nature will eventually take its course. This is opposed to interventionist obstetrics, which aims at medical technological intervention. Although it is traditional, today expectative obstetrics is seen as a modern ideal by many women and health professionals.

Prenatal care is available everywhere in the Netherlands to all women, whatever their socio-economic status and income, and consists of an average of twelve visits. It includes counseling about the processes of birth and pregnancy, and about nutrition, as well as prenatal risk assessment to decide which women can have their babies at home,[3] assisted by a midwife or general practitioner, and to refer women with high-risk pregnancies to a fully equipped obstetric department. Because of the easy availability of contraceptives and abortion, the number of unwanted pregnancies is relatively low. As a consequence, most women are motivated to participate in the prenatal programs, which include breathing and relaxation exercises, and believe that the way they prepare to give birth is highly relevant to its outcome.

Contrary to the image of the passive woman, whose clinical delivery is managed by a team of professionals, the practice of home delivery is based on the model of an active woman who retains control of her body and her baby. The woman in childbirth is the main actor, supported by a midwife or general practitioner, and usually by the baby's father or a friend or relative. Close friends, relatives, or neighbors may share the event of birth or come to the house directly afterwards. Birth is considered a family event.

Comparing different obstetric systems, Brigitte Jordan concludes:

> One of the most significant consequences of a system's choice of birth location is that this choice assigns responsibility for the course of labor and credit for its outcome. In hospital deliveries, responsibility and credit are clearly the physicians'. At home, by contrast, the initiative remains in many ways with the woman and her family. The birth is their choice, their problem, their task, and will finally be their achievement.[4]

There is a further issue for which birth location matters, namely the issue of mother-infant separation. If birth location is unmarked and unspecialized, mother and child remain together from the moment of birth. When home birth came under attack in the 1960s and 1970s, it became a highly emotional subject of debate in medical circles, as well as among health-care consumers, especially prospective parents. Although doctors have focused on whether a relationship exists between perinatal mortality and morbidity rates and place of delivery, many parents also emphasize the quality of care and the experience of women and families of the birth event. Giving birth is viewed as a rich and valuable experience, and a woman's feelings of pride and satisfaction over a successful birth are viewed as an optimal basis for her relationship with the child. In the 1980s, conferences and other meetings that were open to the general public drew large crowds eager to collect information on all details of pregnancy and birth. They were unanimous in their support of home birth and the belief that to maintain it, continuous vigilance is necessary.

Analgesics are rarely employed. These are considered unnecessary for a normal birth. The use of chloroform to make delivery less painful, which came into vogue with Queen Victoria in 1853, and "Twilight Sleep," which was developed in nearby Germany and became popular in the United States after 1915,[5] were never introduced in the Netherlands. Medication has not become part of the cultural definition of normal deliveries, and this view has influenced the attitudes of Dutch women. The great majority does not expect medication. Comparing medicated and nonmedicated deliveries in four countries, Jordan suggests that women's expectations influence the level of pain displayed and experienced.[6] This is in agreement with the observations of Mark Zborowski[7] on the impact of culture on the experience and expression of pain. Although in the 1920s American women campaigned for hospitalization and painless birth under anesthesia, Dutch women have never openly expressed such views. Before World War II, politically active women's groups only showed concern for the health of babies;[8] since the 1970s, however, feminists have been in favor of home deliveries assisted by a midwife.

MIDWIVES AND MATERNITY HOME-CARE ASSISTANTS

Midwives together with general practitioners are responsible for attending all normal home and hospital births. Midwives resist the medicalization of birth and pregnancy (Abraham in this volume). They give full attention to the social and psychological aspects of these processes, and employ only low medical technology, compared to the high medical technology that is available in the obstetric departments of hospitals. There is, however, a minority of midwives who are in favor of introducing more medical technology into their practice (Tymstra in this volume). The high percentage of home births is directly related to the decision made in 1941 by the *Ziekenfondsen*, the system of Dutch national health insurance that covers 65 percent of the population, to give midwives a monopoly over normal obstetrics. It was argued that their training and experience made midwives more expert at normal deliveries than the average medical practitioner. The monopoly implies that in normal home deliveries, the insurance pays for the services of a midwife, which include all prenatal and postnatal care. A general practitioner may be called in if no midwife is available in the municipality. Hospitalization used to be covered only where there was some suspicion or evidence of a problem. Since the 1980s, however, women covered by the *Ziekenfondsen* (national health insurance) who prefer the twenty-four-hour or short-stay hospital delivery to home birth are reimbursed. Women who have private insurance are free to choose between home and hospital delivery, and between the services of a midwife or a general practitioner.

Pregnant women can consult a midwife directly rather than seeing a doctor first. Women with complicated pregnancies and/or deliveries are referred to obstetricians, and as a rule, give birth in hospitals. In the 1990s, the midwives' monopoly is a matter of debate, since radical reorganization of the national health insurance is being prepared.[9]

In 1990, one-third of all babies were born at home, whereas the mothers of another third opted for a short-stay hospital delivery, which is a stay in the hospital of twenty-four hours at most. The mother is attended by a primary health-care professional, either a midwife or general practitioner, and spends the lying-in period at home. The short-stay hospital delivery was introduced in 1965 and soon became popular. It is a compromise between what many women perceive as the "safety" of hospital birth and the domesticity of home birth (van Daalen in this volume).

Giving birth at home and spending the lying-in period at home are made possible by the maternity home-care assistant (van Teijlingen in this volume). The maternity home-care assistant helps the midwife during delivery and gives postnatal care, supervised by the midwife. Her work enables the latter to dedicate herself fully to medical and social tasks.

Midwives consider the maternity home-care assistant as indispensable. Apart from helping during delivery, the assistant takes care of mother and child (up to eight hours per day) during the first seven to eight days after delivery, and may also perform all necessary chores in the household. Moreover, she functions as a coach for the mother. Midwife Astrid Limburg states that women who give birth at home become more easily self-confident mothers, because they have been with their babies continuously and know their behavior intimately. The Netherlands is the only country where promoting the well-being of mother and child during the lying-in period is attended to by the State. The World Health Organization comments that the way this service is organized makes the Netherlands the envy of all the other European countries.[10] However, because of cuts in government spending, maternity home-care assistance is being threatened. In the big cities, the service is no longer functioning optimally because of lack of funds and personnel.

THE PLACE OF BIRTH

The Nineteenth Century

Hospital deliveries were introduced in the nineteenth century. Before then, the hospitals (*gasthuizen*) that were financed by the towns to serve the poor and destitute did not admit women about to give birth, according to a decree of 1687. In 1828, "clinical schools" (Marland in this volume) were opened in Amsterdam and Rotterdam based on the model of institutions that already existed in France, Austria, and Germany. Because the houses of the poor were not judged suitable for instruction, doctors taught midwives, surgeons, and medical students in these "schools." Poor women were given free treatment and were even paid a small fee to deliver at the clinic so students could gain practical experience. The lying-in period was to be spent at home.[11] It was emphasized that no form of coercion should be used to hospitalize pregnant women, as clinical delivery was considered contrary to the Dutch national character. For example, in 1826, the Rotterdam City Council stated:

> The knowledge and experience that we have of our countrymen's customs and mentality make us consider ... that a maternal ward is absolutely contrary to our national character, and that no woman, no matter how humble her descent, might be prepared to put up with a total separation from all her kin and relations. We strongly doubt whether, in case it would be possible to induce women to submit to this remedy, their husband and other relatives would agree.... We tremble ... when we think of the pain and distress of the sufferers who, no matter how low they may have fallen, have to endure being the subject of education for young students.[12]

The "clinical schools" or lying-in hospitals established to provide facilities for clinical education did not become popular. In the clinics of Amsterdam and Rotterdam, conditions of hygiene and general care were deplorable, and the rates of maternal and infant death high (Hiddinga in this volume). In 1865, the clinical schools were replaced by training colleges for midwives in Amsterdam and Rotterdam (Marland in this volume). Even then, in the maternity ward of the Amsterdam municipal hospital, asepsis and antisepsis were absent until a new director (Van der Mey) introduced them in 1880. His predecessor (Lehman), who had been director for thirty years, had been an opponent of such practices. During Van der Mey's management, maternal deaths from puerperal fever dropped, and infant mortality decreased by 50 percent.[13]

M. J. Van Lieburg and Hilary Marland point out that the lack of institutional facilities ensured that most women, rich or poor, continued to have their babies at home.[14] They mention that around 1900 the very low incidence of hospital births was one of the main features that set the practice of obstetrics in the Netherlands apart from other countries, in particular from

England and the United States, where the number of lying-in clinics and obstetric wards in hospitals was increasing. Hospitalization became significant
only after World War II, and as late as 1960, 74 percent of babies were born
at home.[15]

Medicalization in the 1960s and 1970s

With the exception of a short period following World War II, throughout the
twentieth century birth rates dropped in all Western industrialized countries
except for the Netherlands. There, change did not come until the 1960s. In
1952, for example, the birth rate was 22.8 in the Netherlands, higher than
Ireland's 21.8.[16] It was only surpassed in Europe by Portugal (24.7) and was
described as a "demographic anomaly."[17] The high birth rates in the 1940s
and 1950s had an impact on the relations between midwives and general
practitioners. Because there were plenty of deliveries to attend, rivalry between the two groups was muted. In the years that followed, however, change
in birthing practices accelerated. Since the 1960s, medicalization increased,
while the birth rate dropped dramatically, and the number of midwives, obstetricians, and general practitioners started to rise. Between 1972 and 1982,
midwives increased 12 percent, general practitioners 22, and obstetricians
64.[18] This has resulted in considerable changes in the division of labor among
them.[19] Hospital deliveries attended by obstetricians have increased rapidly,
whereas the percentage of deliveries done by midwives remains more or less
the same, and the general practitioners have lost ground. The number of general practitioners attending deliveries is decreasing annually. The percentage
of home deliveries dropped dramatically, from 74 percent in 1960 to 44 percent in 1975 and 36 percent in 1978. From 1978 to 1985, it remained relatively stable, fluctuating between 35 and 37 percent. Since 1985, however, it
shows a slight decline.[20]

The hospitalization of birth started in the cities, and today the place of delivery (home versus hospital) is still related to urbanization. In small communities, the percentages of births taking place at home are much larger than in
the urban centers. Towns with more than 100,000 inhabitants have more
hospital deliveries (including short-stay hospital deliveries). In general, regional differences are striking and show that a high percentage of hospital deliveries is, among other things, related to the presence of a teaching
hospital.[21]

Prenatal Risk Assessment and the Place of Birth

During prenatal care, midwives and general practitioners determine which
women have pathological pregnancies, as well as those cases at risk for pathology (Treffers in this volume). These must be referred to an obstetrician.
Cases of apparent obstetrical or medical pathology that cannot be solved dur-

ing pregnancy fall into the category "medical indication for hospitalization." All in this category must be hospitalized for their delivery, which must be supervised by an obstetrician.

To limit the increasing hospitalization, in 1973 the national health insurance system introduced a list of medical indications (Treffers in this volume) to distinguish between normal (physiological) and complicated (pathological) deliveries. This list, known as the Kloosterman list, was developed by Dr. Gerrit-Jan Kloosterman (interview in this volume). It has been used by midwives and doctors as a guideline for hospitalization, and has been revised a number of times.

As medical technology advanced, examinations and diagnoses became more refined, fewer risks were taken, and more and more women were put in the category of "medical indication." Nationally, medical indications increased rapidly, from 15 percent in 1970 to 45 percent in 1988.[22] Although the majority of obstetricians favor home birth attended by a midwife, there are also advocates of hospitalization. The growing medicalization of birth affects hospitals, health insurance, medical personnel, and last but not least women and their families. In brief, its consequences are economic, as well as social and psychological.

Of course, apart from growing medicalization, there are other explanations for the increase in hospital delivery. These include the age at which women bear their first child. Today they are generally older (the average age at which Dutch women had their first baby was 27.5 in 1989, compared to 23.4 in 1960). Moreover, families are smaller (the average number of children per woman was 1.62 in 1990, compared to 3.1 in 1960),[23] so there is a larger percentage of first-born babies, with a higher risk associated with first deliveries.

Yet policy makers, midwives, some doctors, and some parents objected to the increase in medical indications and its iatrogenic effects. It was also pointed out that a medical indication is financially advantageous, because it entitles the woman to have the delivery and stay in the hospital free of charge. Referrals were sometimes based on the doctor's or woman's personal preference. Today this is more difficult.

In 1983, because of dissatisfaction with the increasing medicalization of birth, the government again convened a working group to revise the Kloosterman list. For this working group, as well as for the government-appointed Committee for Advice on Obstetrical Care, home birth is the norm. At present, the new list of medical indications, which was drawn up in 1987, provides the guidelines for determining when midwives and general practitioners (who take care of normal births) should be in charge and when the services of obstetricians (who are responsible for pathological births) should be employed. The emphasis is on allocating medical expertise where it is most beneficial, namely, in the treatment of cases that clearly fall within the medical domain. Before 1987, if an obstetrical or medical problem was detected during prenatal screening for risk, midwives would refer the woman to an obstetrician. In some cases, even if a doctor was able to solve the problem, he might not send the woman back to the midwife. Rather, he would book her for hospital delivery. The revision of 1987 (Working Group Revision Kloosterman) recognizes three categories of pregnancies: low risk (eligible for home delivery), high risk (hospital delivery), and medium risk. The midwife sends women in the medium-risk category to an obstetrician for a consultation, after which the midwife decides whether to keep the woman under her care or refer her definitely to the obstetrician. Many midwives do not view the revision as changing their basically satisfactory working relationships with obstetricians. Nevertheless, the revision does give the midwife a considerable amount of decision-making power: She is now formally entitled to categorize normal and abnormal pregnancies, and she is the one who makes the final decision.

On the basis of her research findings, Martine Eskes states that the new list of medical indications in itself is satisfactory, but that its successful application depends on the cooperation of midwives, general practitioners, and obstetricians.[24] The aim of the 1987 revision of the selection system is to limit the power of general practitioners and obstetricians to regulate the flow of hospital deliveries, reduce the number of unnecessary medical indications, and enhance greater consensus in decision making among practitioners. The revision has, however, caused a considerable amount of disagreement among the three occupational groups, with obstetricians especially objecting to midwives' newly acquired decision-making power.[25]

One might argue that to a certain extent the model of home delivery is a middle-class model. When Kloosterman's list of medical indications for hospitalization was introduced in 1973, a "social" indication was added. Those women living in poor housing and, in general, those whose lifestyle is too deviant from middle-class values, may be given a "social" indication for hospitalization. From 1948 to 1970 in Amsterdam, women in this category gave birth in the Zeeburg Unit that was attached to the University of Amsterdam. Since the revision of the list in 1987, the former "social" indication for hospitalization includes women using hard drugs, those with psychiatric problems, and those who plan to give their babies up for adoption.[26]

Perinatal Mortality and the Place of Birth

Since 1955, the Dutch perinatal mortality rate has no longer been the lowest in the world. The rate decreased continuously but somewhat slower than in the Scandinavian countries. In the 1970s, the statistics on perinatal mortality of the various countries sparked off a debate about whether the Netherlands should follow the example of other European countries that had chosen complete hospitalization, or whether the traditional Dutch system with a high percentage of home deliveries should be preserved and improved.

In 1978 Kloosterman's article "Obstetrics in the Netherlands: the parting of ways" in the *Dutch Journal of Medicine* (*Nederlands Tijdschrift voor Geneeskunde*)[27] provoked a passionate polemic that lasted from January 1978 until May 1979, when the editors of the journal stopped it. The debate centered on the risks and safety of home delivery versus hospital delivery. In response to Kloosterman's plea for the preservation of home delivery, opponents presented statistics supporting a causal relationship between hospital delivery and the decrease in perinatal mortality. In other words, statistics from 1952–75 were interpreted to show that increased hospital deliveries led to decreased perinatal mortality. However, a statistical relationship is not necessarily indicative of a causal relationship: Cause-and-effect arguments were shown to be spurious and were defeated on logical grounds.[28]

A survey carried out by S. Damstra-Wijmenga in 1982[29] showed that home delivery is characterized by low perinatal mortality and little medical intervention (actually, the latter was also emphasized in 1911 by Dr. Catharina van Tussenbroek).[30] In a later publication Damstra-Wijmenga concluded that research has not proven that home birth is associated with any higher perinatal mortality than clinical delivery (see Buitendijk in this volume).[31] She warned that further medicalization may result in an increase in infant mortality because of iatrogenic and nosocomial effects.[32]

The debate was taken up in the *British Journal of Obstetrics and Gynaecology* (July 1986) with articles on the place of delivery in the Netherlands, Denmark, and England. In that issue, P. E. Treffers and R. Laan state that the proportion of hospital deliveries does not appear to be a major factor in the perinatal mortality rate in the current system of obstetric care in the Netherlands.[33] Their conclusion is based on a study carried out in the twelve provinces of the country. Sicco Scherjon, who presents a comparison of the organization of obstetrics in the Netherlands and Denmark, reaches the same conclusion as Treffers and Laan: the slower decrease in the Dutch perinatal mortality rate compared with the Danish rate cannot be explained by the high proportion of Dutch home deliveries.[34] They emphasize that perinatal mortality rates of different countries are not fully comparable, and R. Campbell and A. Macfarlane point out: "It is . . . inappropriate to use crude perinatal mortality rates as indicators of the quality of maternity care."[35] A working group of the World Health Organization found that criteria for the Standard Perinatal Mortality are applied differently in different countries (Buitendijk in this volume).

Moreover, there are several nonmedical factors that have an impact on perinatal mortality, such as the general welfare of a population, dietary patterns, and various demographic factors. Yet, when in 1986 D. Hoogendoorn published an article on perinatal mortality and the place of birth in the *Dutch Journal of Medicine* (*Nederlands Tijdschrift voor Geneeskunde*), the polemic of 1978–79 was repeated, along with the same arguments (Buitendijk, this volume).[36]

In the study carried out by Eskes, the results of the selection system (list of medical indications) were evaluated with respect to infant mortality and morbidity and the place of birth, at home, in the maternity unit, in a hospital under the supervision of a midwife, or in a hospital under the care of an obstetrician.[37] Eskes is not in favor of reorganizing the existing system of obstetric care. The outcome of her research is that healthy women who have their babies at home and are attended by midwives have fewer risks from unnecessary medical diagnosis and intervention.

Although in the debate on perinatal mortality different models of giving birth are evaluated in medical terms, attention to the value of the birth experience for women and their families is not absent. Various doctors who favor home birth stress the importance of birth as a family event, and some of them even assume that home birth is an intrinsic part of Dutch national character.[38]

The Family and Home Birth

Home birth fits in the picture of the domesticity (van Daalen in this volume) and introversion described as characteristic of traditional Dutch family life in the middle and upper classes. Donald Haks emphasizes the traditional autonomy of the Dutch conjugal family.[39] He concludes that the nuclear or conjugal family was the basic unit of the Dutch kinship system as early as the seventeenth and eighteenth centuries, and points out that this unit showed many modern characteristics: there were relatively few contacts with kin outside the nuclear cell, there was free choice of partner based upon mutual affection, and there was a certain degree of equality and intimacy between spouses and among parents and children. Haks describes the well-to-do family of the seventeenth and eighteenth centuries as particularly home- and child-oriented. Simon Schama sketches a similar picture: "With the birth of a child, the happy family entered a sort of state of civic grace . . . the birth was very much a semi-public and neighborhood event, with innumerable parties and feasts marking the earliest calendar of the child."[40]

Writing about the 1960s, Johan Goudsblom states: "If there are any distinct Dutch national character traits, these are likely to be nourished in the family." "Privacy, concern for respectability, orderliness, discretion, seclusiveness" are traits of the "strongly introverted family culture." "Great value is attached to family cohesion; birthdays and wedding anniversaries are regularly observed."[41] The event of birth itself can also be looked upon as one of the high points of social life. Regardless of the radical changes in the family since the 1960s, this is still true today.[42] The majority of women have only one or two children, which increases the value attached to the birth experience.

CONCLUDING OBSERVATIONS

Government policies have shown consistent support for home birth. Moreover, the State has made severe cuts in the costs of health care, which favors the less expensive services of midwives. But cost is only one factor in this matter. Home birth is considered a valuable cultural pattern that must be safeguarded. In the 1980s, the Dutch model of home birth has received attention from the World Health Organization, as well as at international conferences on obstetrics and meetings for the general public. In 1986, at a large meeting devoted to birthing practices in Amsterdam, the English advocate of home delivery, Sheila Kitzinger, stated: "The Dutch are ahead of us." But they are ahead because, in the twentieth century, the process of medicalization developed later and at a slower rate in the Netherlands. In the past twenty years, although the medicalization of birth has definitely increased, it has not become pervasive. State support, midwives' advanced professionalization, their powerful organization, increasing popularity, and the support received from various obstetricians all help to maintain the high regard for home birth. Also important are the increased assertiveness of health consumers, the increased criticism of medical practitioners by the women's movement, and criticism of the medicalization of delivery along with praise for the Dutch model of home birth in various countries. Referring to England, Ann Oakley mentions a "consumer's revolt" and the implementation of alternative services.[43] This is also true for the United States. Although the movement of home birth supporters is new, for a Dutch woman, having babies at home is traditional.[44] It appears that feminism has given this tradition a new impulse. In the urban centers, the choice for home birth is most prevalent among highly educated middle-class women.[45] The highest percentages of home deliveries are, however, still found in the rural parts of the country, where the continuity with the past remains important. Kloosterman stated that, although significant progress has been made in obstetrics and infant care, the definition given by the Dutch obstetrician Hendrik van Deventer in 1701 still holds today: "A natural birth is a birth accomplished by Nature alone, without any help or Art, and in which no artificial help from midwives or men midwives is needed, that is, until the very moment of birth or delivery."[46]

Treffers and Laan emphasize that today the good quality of home delivery in the Netherlands may not be automatically transferable outside the country.[47] It must be considered in the context of the Dutch situation, including highly qualified midwives, good prenatal and postnatal care, maternity home-care assistants, a careful system for screening high- and low-risk pregnancies, the high density of hospitals, and the absence of isolated rural areas (if complications suddenly occur during a delivery at home, rapid transport to a nearby hospital is easy).

Yet, although the social context in which birth is embedded and the cultural experience surrounding it differ from one country to the other, the Dutch model is relevant for other countries (Katz Rothman in this volume). Eva Albermann observes, in her commentary on research on the place of birth in the Netherlands, the United Kingdom, and Denmark, that "all the available evidence suggests that in carefully selected and well-supervised low-risk deliveries the extra risk for mother and baby attributable only to the absence of hospital facilities is low, and the satisfaction of a successful delivery high."[48] Writing about England, Albermann points out that if the expense of a sizeable domiciliary service is considered too high, it is necessary for hospitals to make available the type of low-technology care that many of their clients prefer. This may be an unsatisfactory compromise, however, since research shows that hospital deliveries, chosen by women without any medical problems and intended to be low tech, have considerably higher rates of medical intervention than home births (both Treffers and Buitendijk in this volume).

Today in most Western industrialized societies, giving birth is defined as a medical event. In the Netherlands, however, the medicalization of pregnancy and birthing started later, and even when it finally gained some acceptance, it met strong resistance and developed more slowly. The division of labor between obstetricians and midwives, and the accommodation between high and low medical technology that goes with it, resulted in the unique Dutch situation. The Dutch pattern is related to the organization of obstetrics that has developed, and in particular, the autonomous position of midwives in it. Behind this pattern is an ideology that places a high value on motherhood and the home.

Not all is well, however. The present Dutch system of home birth and midwifery is in flux and should not be taken for granted. In the near future, the system of national health insurance will be radically reorganized, and one of the main characteristics of the new system will be a limitation of the role played by the government and an increase of the responsibilities and empowerment of consumers, insurers, and providers of health care (individuals as well as institutions). It is not certain whether under the new system the midwives will be able to maintain their legal monopoly over normal obstetrics. Neither is the maintenance of maternity home care secured. Moreover, the rapid advance of medical technology for prenatal diagnosis, considered as progress by some and a threat by others, cannot be ignored (see both Katz Rothman and Tymstra in this volume). In the coming years, it will definitely have an impact for midwifery. Finally, there is a shortage of midwives. The future of home birth and midwifery is in the balance.

The chapters of this anthology examine the functioning and development of the Dutch model of home birthing and midwifery. Marland sheds light on the way midwifery evolved and deals with the debate concerning the competence of midwives around the turn of the century, based largely on the various reports and accompanying discussions that appeared in medical and midwives' journals.

Anja Hiddinga pictures the slow development of Dutch obstetrics in the nineteenth century. Compared to their German colleagues, Dutch obstetricians emphasized education and practical work, and did little scientific research. She relates this historical development to "the critical and relativizing

attitude towards new therapies and widely announced medical achievements"
that today still exist among obstetricians who support home birth.

Rineke van Daalen suggests that the preference of many Dutch women for
home birth is related to the history of the Dutch family from the seventeenth
century on. She does this by analyzing written sources as well as pictures and
paintings.

Pieter Treffers explains the selection system for normal and complicated
deliveries that is the basis for decision making on the place of birth, as well as
the division of labor between midwives and obstetricians. This system is crucial in the unique Dutch accommodation of high and low obstetric technology.

Simone Buitendijk deals with polemics about the implications of the course
of the Dutch perinatal mortality rate since the 1950s, and discusses the medical literature on the safety of home births in the Netherlands, as well as elsewhere. Tjeerd Tymstra warns that the increased use of highly developed
medical technology for prenatal diagnosis is in conflict with the concept of
pregnancy as a normal physiological process and endangers midwives' low-
technology approach.

Eva Abraham gives an overview of midwifery. Since the seventeenth century, it evolved differently from the way it developed in the other European
countries. In the twentieth century, Dutch midwives became autonomous
medical professionals. Yet they employ only low medical technology.

Edwin van Teijlingen makes clear how maternity home-care assistants play
a crucial role in making home birth accessible to all Dutch women. L. H.
Lumey highlights the role of the State by comparing the arguments about
home birth given by a number of government committees in the Netherlands
and the United Kingdom. Rineke van Daalen and Reinie van Goor contribute
an interview with Dr. G. J. Kloosterman, who has played a leading role in
shaping the present Dutch obstetric model. Finally, Barbara Katz Rothman
deals with the implications of the Dutch obstetric system for those of other
countries, in particular the United States.

NOTES

1. Of all deliveries 33.4 percent take place at home, 33 percent are clinical (delivery and lying-in period occur at the hospital), and 32 percent are short-stay hospital deliveries. Hessing-Wagner, J. C., *Geboorte en zorgverniewing* (Rijswijk: Sociaal en
Cultureel Planbureau, 1991).

2. Jordan, Brigitte, *Birth in Four Cultures* (Montreal: Eden Press Women's Publications, 1978): 43–44.

3. "A woman meets the requirements for home delivery if she is in good health,
with no symptoms of toxemia, no fetopelvic disproportion (the head of the infant has
descended in the last few weeks of pregnancy or at least can be brought into contact
with the small pelvis), has a single fetus, no abnormalities in her medical history (except one or two uncomplicated early abortions), is younger than 35 with no previous

births, or younger than 40 with previous births, and experiencing spontaneous labor after the 37th week and before the end of the 42nd week. The expectant mother must have a heated bedroom at home and it must be possible to transfer her to a hospital within half an hour." Kloosterman, quoted in Eskes, M., *Het Wormerveer onderzoek: Meerjarenonderzoek naar de kwaliteit van de verloskundige zorg rond een vroedvrouwenpraktijk*, (1989): 243. Fifteen percent of all women who are booked for home delivery are transferred to a hospital during labor. The country's small size and the high density of hospitals make this feasible.

4. Jordan, 1978: 50.

5. Wertz, Dorothy and Richard Wertz, *Lying-In, A History of Childbirth in America* (New York: The Free Press, 1977): 150–154.

6. Jordan, 1978, pp. 35–37.

7. Zborowski, Mark, "Cultural components in responses to pain," *Journal of Social Issues* 8 (4) (1952): 16–30; and Zborowski, Mark, *People in Pain* (San Francisco: Jossey-Bass, 1969).

8. van Daalen, Rineke, "The state of infant health care in Amsterdam: Medicalization and the role of the state," *Netherlands Journal of Sociology*, 21 (2) (October 1985): 126–140.

9. Hessing-Wagner, 1991.

10. World Health Organization, *Having a Baby in Europe* (Copenhagen: World Health Organization, 1985).

11. Van Lieburg, M. J., "Het verloskundig onderwijs aan de klinische school (1828–1867)," in *1882–1982, Rijkskweekschool voor Vroedvrouwen te Rotterdam*, Scholte, E., M. J. Van Lieburg, and R. O. Aalbersberg (eds.) (Leidschendam: Ministerie van Volksgezondheid en Milieuhygiene, 1982): 21–40.

12. Ibid., 22.

13. Verdoorn, J. A., *Het gezondheidswezen te Amsterdam in de 19e eeuw* (Nijmegen: SUN, 1981).

14. Van Lieburg, M. J., and Hilary Marland, "Midwife regulation, education, and practice in the Netherlands during the nineteenth century," *Medical History*, 33 (1989): 296–317.

15. van Daalen, "De groei van de ziekenhuisbevalling, Nederland en het buitenland," *Amsterdams Sociologisch Tijdschrift*, 15 (3) (1988): 414–445.

16. In the 1960s, the exceptionally high Dutch birth rates were the subject of a debate between two Dutch sociologists, Hofstee and Van Heek. Hofstee argued that the same decline in birth rate that took place in other countries operated also in the Netherlands, but at a different pace, especially in the southern and eastern parts of the country. He emphasized the slowness of change in traditional norms and values about the family in those regions. The very essence of what he called the traditional mentality was its resistance to change. Hofstee, E. W., "De groei van de Nederlandse bevolking," *Drift en Koers: een halve eeuw sociale verandering in Nederland*, in: den Hollander, A.N.J. (ed.) (Assen: Van Gorcum, 1961); and Hofstee, E. W., "Het proces der geboortedaling in Nederland, 1850–1960," in Heeren, H. J. and Ph.van Praag (eds.), *Van nu tot nul*, 36–75. (Utrecht/Antwerpen: Het Spectrum, 1963).

Van Heek focused on the differential birth rates of various religious groups and on the great zeal of the Roman Catholics as a disadvantaged minority group fighting for their emancipation in a Calvinistic country since the end of the nineteenth century

(Van Heek, F., *Het geboorte-niveau der Nederlandse Rooms-Katholieken, Een demografisch-sociologische studie van een geemancipeerde minderheidsgroep* [Leiden: Stenfert Kroese, 1963]). The Roman Catholic birth rate remained considerably higher than that of the Protestants (except for the fundamentalist *Gereformeerden*). It was also higher than the birth rate of their co-religionists just across the border, in Belgium and Germany. Van Heek pointed out that the Roman Catholics displayed a remarkable religious élan and fighting spirit, and that the "*lutte des berceaux*" (having large families as a weapon) has been one of the means in their struggle. He stated that it was also a direct effect of strict obedience to religious mandates concerning reproduction and that it cannot be denied that even in the 1950s the Dutch priests were praising the creation of very large families as a work pleasing to God. It was indeed seen as the proper task of priests to remind couples of their duty to procreate. Moreover, not only did the Roman Catholics have an effectively organized system of social control over their followers, but they were also successful in pressing the national government to stimulate a social climate that favored the family as a crucial institution. Thus, the Roman Catholic and the socialist political parties joined forces to pass laws that strongly supported a generous scheme of family subsidies, with progressive rates for larger families (William Petersen, 1955). The Roman Catholics were concentrated in the poor southern and eastern parts of the country that Hofstee had classified as traditional and resistant to change. The explanations of Hofstee and Van Heek reinforce one another. Moreover, in later publications, Hofstee recognized the direct influence confessional groups had on the birth rates of the 1950s (Hofstee, E. W., 1 *Korte demografische geschiedenis van Nederland van 1800 tot heden* (Haarlem: Fibula-Van Dishoeck, 1981).

17. Petersen, William, "Family subsidies in the Netherlands," *Marriage and Family Living*, XVII, (1955): 260–266.

18. Butter, I., and E. M. Lapré, "Verloskundige zorg in Nederland," *Economisch Sociale Berichten* (January 15, 1986): 425–431.

19. In 1990, 45 percent of all deliveries were attended by midwives, 11 percent by general practitioners, and 44 percent by (or supervised by) obstetricians. Hessing-Wagner, 1991.

20. *Tachtig jaren statistiek in tijdreeksen 1899–1979* (The Hague: Staatsuitgeverij, 1979); Hessing-Wagner, 1991.

21. Hessing-Wagner, J. C., *Samenhang in de zorg rond geboorte en jonge kinderen* (Rijswijk: Sociaal en Cultureel Planbureau, 1985).

22. Centraal Bureau voor de Statistiek, 1991.

23. Klinkert, J. J., *Verloskundigen en artsen* (Alphen a.d.Rijn: Stafleu's Wetenschappelijke Uitgeversmij, 1980).

24. Eskes, Martine, *Het Wormerveer Onderzoek, meerjarenonderzoek naar de kwaliteit van de verloskundige zorg rond een vroedvrouwenpraktijk* (Wormerveer, no publisher, 1989).

25. Riteco, J. A., and L. Hingstman, *Evaluatie Invoering 'Verloskundige Indicatielijst.'* Utrecht, Nederlands Instituut voor Onderzoek van de Eerstelijnsgezondheiszorg (NIVEL) (1991): 114–116.

26. Ridderbeek, T.J.J., "Bevallingen en kraamzorg, GE 1987/1988." *Maandbericht Gezondheid*, 12 (1990): 4–13.

27. Kloosterman, G. J., "Verloskunde in Nederland op de Tweesprong" (Obstetrics

in the Netherlands: the parting of the ways), *Nederlands Tijdschrift voor Geneeskunde*, 122 (23) (1978): 1161–1170.

28. In a debate in England about the relationship between hospitalization and infant mortality, with similar data and conclusions (*Department of Health and Social Security*, 1976), the same error was made. Cochrane said about this case: "every student knows this sort of correlation is not evidence," adding that it is similar to the high correlation between perinatal mortality and average length of postnatal stay in the hospital. Cochrane, A., *Effectiveness and efficiency, random reflections on health services* (Abingdon: Nuffield Provincial Hospitals Trusts, 1972).

29. Damstra-Wijmenga, S., *Veilig Bevallen, een vergelijkende studie tussen de thuisbevalling en de klinische bevalling* (Groningen, no publisher, 1982).

30. Van Tusschenbroek, Catharina, *De ontwikkeling der aseptische verloskunde in Nederland* (Haarlem: De Erven F. Bohn, 1911).

31. Damstra-Wijmenga, S., "1982 and Perinatale Sterfte en Thuisbevalling," in *Vorderingen en Praktijk*, Mulder, J. D. (ed.) (Leiden: Rijksuniversiteit, Boerhaave Commissie voor Postacademisch Onderzoek in de Geneeskunde, 1986).

32. Iatrogenic effects are those resulting from treatment by a physician; nosocomial effects are those originating in a hospital.

33. Treffers, P. E., and R. Laan, "Regional perinatal mortality and regional hospitalization at delivery in the Netherlands," *British Journal of Obstetrics and Gynaecology*, 93 (July 1986): 190–193.

34. Scherjon, Sicco, "A comparison between the organization of obstetrics in Denmark and the Netherlands," *British Journal of Obstetrics and Gynaecology*, 93 (July 1986): 684–689.

35. Campbell, R., and A. Macfarlane, "Place of delivery: a review," *British Journal of Obstetrics and Gynaecology*, 93 (July 1986): 675–683.

36. Hoogendoorn, D., "Indrukwekkende en tegelijk teleurstellende daling van de perinatale sterfte in Nederland," in *Nederlands Tijdschrift voor Geneeskunde*, 130 (32) (1986): 1436–1440.

37. Eskes, 1989.

38. Sikkel, A., "Epiloog," in Scholte, Van Lieburg, Aalbersberg (1982): 200.

39. Haks, Donald, *Huwelijk en gezin in Holland in de 17de en 18de eeuw* (Assen: Van Gorcum, 1982).

40. Schama, Simon, *The Embarrassment of Riches* (New York: Knopf, 1987).

41. Goudsblom, Johan, *Dutch Society* (New York: Random House, 1968).

42. One aspect of the Dutch cult of domesticity has been the comparatively low percentages of employed women. The industrialization process started late, after 1870, and did not require as many women as in England or other Western countries because of the availability of sufficient male workers. Moreover, those women in the lower social classes who were employed had to face deplorable working conditions and, at the end of the nineteenth century, high maternal mortality was found among them (Schilstra, W. N., 1940, *Vrouwenarbeid en Industrie in Nederland in de tweede helft der Negentiende eeuw.* Nijmegen: SUN-reprint, 1976). When better social conditions allowed these women to stay at home, many adopted the domesticity of the middle classes (de Regt, Ali, 1984, *Arbeidersgezinnen en beschavingsarbeid, ontwikkelingen in Nederland 1870–1940*, Meppel: Boom). Although this trend changed in the 1960s, percentages of employed women today are lower than those of the

other countries of the European Community. Various authors (Bots, Mirre, and Maria Noordman, *Moederschap als balsem*, Amsterdam: SUA, 1981; Grunell, Marianne, *Thuis in de jaren vijftig*, Amsterdam: SUA, 1985) have described the preoccupation with household and motherhood during the 1950s, whereas others have dealt with the changes in women's roles and options in the 1960s and 1970s (Brinkgreve, Christien, and M. Korzec, *Margriet weet raad. Gevoel, gedrag, en moraal in Nederland, 1938–1978*, Utrecht/Antwerpen: Het spectrum, 1978).

43. Oakley, Ann, *The Captured Womb: A History of the Medical Care of Pregnant Women* (Oxford: Basil Blackwell Publisher Ltd., 1984).

44. Katz Rothman, Barbara, *Recreating Motherhood, Ideology and Technology in a Patriarchal Society* (New York: W. W. Norton & Company, 1989).

45. Kleiverda, G., A. M. Steen, I. Andersen, P. E. Treffers, and E. Everaerd, "Place of delivery in the Netherlands: Maternal motives and background variables related to preferences for home or hospital confinement," in *European Journal of Obstetrics, Gynaecology and Reproductive Biology*, 36 (1990): 1–9.

46. Kloosterman, G., "De verloskunde in Vrouw Schrader's 'Memoryboeck,'" in *C. G. Schrader's Memoryboeck van de Vrouwens* (Amsterdam: Rodopi, 1984): 47–80.

47. Treffers, P. E., and R. Laan, pp. 190–193.

48. Albermann, Eva, "The place of birth," *British Journal of Obstetrics and Gynaecology*, 93 (July 1986): 657–658.

I

HISTORICAL BACKGROUND

2

The Guardians of Normal Birth: The Debate on the Standard and Status of the Midwife in the Netherlands around 1900

Hilary Marland

In the 1990s the Dutch system of obstetric care is unique in the Western world for the predominance of midwife-attended births, the high level of home delivery, and the low rate of intervention in the birthing process. Within the Dutch system, the midwife has achieved a large sphere of competence and independence. She (and in recent years to a small extent, he) has secured the task of supervising independently the management of prenatal care, delivery, and postnatal checkups in normal pregnancies and births. Even in cases complicated by medical indications, the midwife, working closely with the obstetrician, may still play a part in caring for the pregnant woman and in the birthing process.[1]

All this is in contrast to the obstetric services that have developed in other Western lands, and is diametrically opposed to the U.S. system, where almost 100 percent of births take place in a hospital. In the United States, births supervised by the obstetrician are often highly medicalized, anesthetics and analgesics are liberally used, and the rate of Caesarean section is about 20 percent, double that of many developed countries.[2] Many see the Dutch system as a model to be followed, because it gives the pregnant woman more choice of where, how, and with whom she will give birth, and the midwife a higher level of professional autonomy. Dutch obstetric services are seen as efficient and economic, and also maintain low rates of perinatal mortality. Thus, it is argued, the Dutch system is highly successful, confirming that "midwives, practising their skills in human relations and without sophisticated technological aids, are the most effective guardians of childbirth and that the emotional security of a familiar setting, the home, makes a greater contribution to

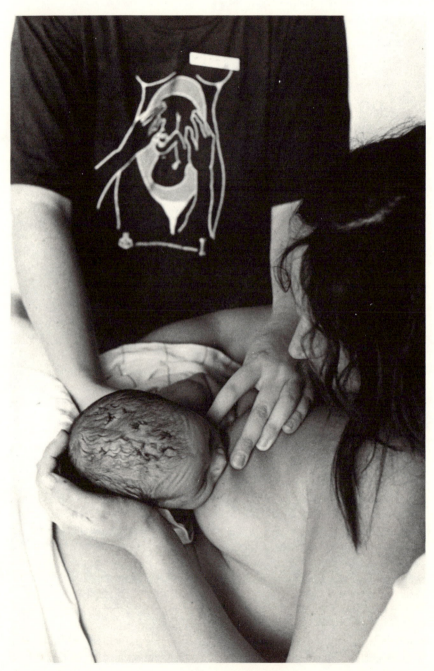

"Aan de Borst Gelegd" ("At the Breast"), 1992. Copyright © by Paul Andriesse.

safety than does the equipment in hospital to facilitate obstetric interventions in cases of emergency."[3]

How did the Dutch system of obstetric care come to differ so much from those of other Western countries? The actual parting of the ways can be placed with some confidence in the twentieth century, though the historical antecedents to this can be traced back to the nineteenth century and still earlier.[4] In most Western countries, the concentration of medical technology in hospitals and maternity clinics began to be a major force in obstetric care from the 1920s and 1930s onwards, stepping up its influence after World War II.[5] The Netherlands was by no means immune to these changes, but their impact was much less in a country where institutionalized births had always been low and hospitalization late compared with other developed countries, and where the midwife continued to manage the majority of normal deliveries.[6]

At the turn of the twentieth century, however, obstetric care in the Netherlands and other Western countries, including the United States, was characterized by similarities as much as contrasts. In the early years of the twentieth century, around 60 percent of births in the Netherlands were midwife-attended, and, at this time, most American babies were also delivered at home by midwives: in 1910, approximately 50 percent.[7] In the United States "hospitalization was impossible for all but the very rich or the charity cases in the wards, obstetricians were few, and general practitioners unreliable."[8] For most Americans, particularly the poor, black, and immigrant populations, birth always took place at home attended by the local midwife. In England, too, the midwife was the most familiar figure at childbirth at the turn of the twentieth century, seconded by the general practitioner; births took place at home, without technological intervention.[9]

Yet it was around 1900 that the question of the midwife's future—if indeed, as many argued, she had one—began to be debated in a number of Western countries. The fierce debate that marked the demise of the midwife in the United States is the best known and documented.[10] It drew the curtain on a process that had been under way for several decades: the rise (but not the maturity) of the specialty of obstetrics, growing dissatisfaction with the midwife, attacks on her competence and suitability to practice, and a desire to shift the scene of birth from the home to institutions, to monitor and intervene in a process regarded increasingly as a state of sickness, abnormality, and danger to the mother and baby. The midwife debate in the United States gives the historian an insight not only into the forces at work in early twentieth-century obstetrics, but also into the status quo in obstetric practice immediately preceding a period of great change.

Though not often characterized as a "midwife debate," the discussion in England surrounding the midwife's future, in particular the question of how and by whom she should be regulated, which finally in 1902, after decades of discussion and pressure group activity, led to the passing of the Midwives Act, not only shows how the winds of change were making their influence felt, but gives us a valuable insight into the status and role of midwives in the late nineteenth century.[11] Analysis of midwife debates indicates how obstetric services and the place of the midwife within these services were likely to develop, revealing the different forces and interests at work. They also give a snapshot of obstetric care—a picture of who was delivering whom, how, and where, at the point when the efficiency and appropriateness of the service, and the midwife's place within it, came into question.

The competence and place of the midwife in Dutch obstetrics were also discussed around the turn of the twentieth century. The debate, an altogether milder affair, without the virulence of the American debate and the endurance of the English, was largely concentrated into two reports drawn up in 1897 and 1911 by the Dutch Society for the Promotion of Medicine (*Nederlandsche Maatschappij tot Bevordering der Geneeskunst, NMG*).[12] These reports give an insight into the midwife's sphere of competence during this period, an indication of the various interests at work within the obstetric service—particularly those of general practitioners and midwives—and a preview of the way in which obstetric services would develop in the future. The second report was reinterpreted and answered in the *Journal for Practical Midwifery* (*Tijdschrift voor Praktische Verloskunde*), the midwives' own platform (albeit one controlled to some extent by its doctor editors), which adds an extra dimension to the debate. This chapter will focus on these reports and the responses to them. It will be shown that it was predictable as early as the turn of the twentieth century that Dutch midwifery would follow a *very* different path from other Western countries. The enduring figure of the Dutch midwife, "the guardian of normal birth," was a guarantor of the continuing importance of home births during the twentieth century.[13]

BACKGROUND

The reports of 1897 and 1911 were grounded in a system of obstetric care that had developed over more than two centuries, from the time when town councils and local medical corporations first attempted to outline and control the work of the midwife in the mid-seventeenth century. During the seventeenth and eighteenth centuries, the larger and more important Dutch towns introduced statutes regulating the practices of local midwives, and set up training courses and examinations to test their competence and suitability to practice.[14] The midwife began to be seen as an important figure in securing safe childbirth and enabling the population to increase. During the eighteenth century, most towns also appointed "municipal midwives" (*stadsvroedvrouwen*), who, for a fixed annual salary, were to deliver poor women without charge. The midwives of Delft, the first group to be regulated in the Netherlands, were brought under the supervision of the surgeons' guild and town council as early as 1656. Midwives working in the town were to submit to the rules and provisions of the surgeons' guild, which would also be responsible for examining midwives and teaching them anatomy. Those passing the examination would receive protection from the guild against women attempting to practice without authorization.

Other towns followed. Amsterdam made the examination of midwives compulsory in 1668, Leiden in 1719, Rotterdam drew up regulations for midwives in 1717, Zwolle in 1757, Groningen in 1766, and Utrecht in 1778. In a few towns, the senior medical men, the "municipal man-midwife" (*stadsvroedmeester*) and members of the medical corporations, gave lessons in midwifery. In Amsterdam, courses were made compulsory in 1679, taught by the anatomist, obstetric doctor, and municipal man-midwife, Frederik Ruysch (1638–1731). In Rotterdam, an ordinance of 1705 instituted special demonstrations in anatomy given by the town lecturer in anatomy, Willem Vink (c. 1680–1763), for aspirant and practicing midwives. In towns with midwife ordinances, expectations concerning the midwife's ability and fitness to practice were similar. Before taking an examination before the surgeons' guild or *Collegium Medicum*, candidates were expected to have attended between ten to sixteen deliveries. On passing the examination and swearing an oath of office, midwives were entitled to hang up a board advertising their profession and, under certain conditions, to practice independently. It was stipulated with great force that in difficult cases of childbirth, the midwife was to call in a man-midwife or surgeon to take over the delivery. Midwives were not permitted to use instruments. As to personal requirements, a minimum age was usually insisted upon. Generally midwives were to be older than twenty-five, though, in fact, they were usually much older. They had to be able to read and write, and, most important, had to have borne children themselves. The regulations drawn up by Willem Vink in Rotterdam in 1717, instructed midwives not to frighten a woman in labor, but rather to calm and comfort her, not to rush or abandon a delivery in order to attend on a richer woman, and instructed midwives to call for the assistance of a surgeon or man-midwife in difficult labors. Some regulations warned against drinking, insisted on cleanliness and neatness, and enjoined midwives not to gossip.

The means of regulating midwives varied from town to town; usually responsibility was shared by the surgeons' guild, *Collegium Medicum* or *Collegium Obstetricum*, and the town council, though in Delft, by the eighteenth century the governors and doctors of the *Gasthuis*, the municipal hospital, had taken charge of controlling midwife practice and appointing municipal midwives. Everywhere the aims were the same: through regulation, to make the midwife answerable to the town authorities, to control her training and practice. If the midwife violated the regulations, she was liable to punitive action, which included a fine, dismissal as municipal midwife, or the removal of her board, the symbol of her craft and authorization to practice. In all the ordinances, emphasis was placed on the need to call for assistance in difficult cases, limiting the work of the midwife to normal births. It was pointed out that such regulations protected the midwife herself against unqualified competitors, and though the regulations also protected and reinforced the power of the medical corporations, during this period of local control it seems that these groups were concerned primarily with supervision of the midwife, rather than seeking to replace her.

It is difficult to make an assessment of the effects of local regulations on midwife practice. Up to and, indeed, throughout the nineteenth century, most midwives were trained solely through apprenticeship to established midwives, and few were able to take advantage of the lessons or anatomy demonstrations given in the towns. The fitness of the municipal doctors to teach these courses could be questioned; few had practical experience of obstetrics, and their study of obstetric texts, anatomical knowledge, and experience of emergency deliveries was not well adapted to the midwife's practice. More significantly, these courses had little more than a marginal impact, reaching very few midwives; the remainder relied on the well-tried though fallible system of apprenticeship and in some cases, a little book learning, which resulted in varied standards of competence. Similarly, many midwives remained outside of the examination and licensing systems set up by the towns; simply by living beyond the town boundaries, they were exempt from the ordinances.

Shining through our blurred view of midwife practice in the early modern period is Vrouw Catharina Schrader (1656–1746), who practiced as a midwife in Friesland, in the north of the country, at the close of the seventeenth century and first half of the eighteenth. A woman of special skills and enormous energy, Vrouw Schrader practiced for many years, from 1693 to 1745 (with an ebb in her work during the years of her second marriage, 1712 to 1720). She attended some 3,060 deliveries up to the age of eighty-eight, all of which she recorded in casebooks, many in considerable detail. Her practice was extraordinarily successful; she recorded a maternal mortality rate of only 4.6 per 1,000 births, and a perinatal morality of 54 per 1,000. Her experience grew as she practiced, a process we can trace in her casebook notes. Early mistakes were acted upon and rectified, her techniques and special skills developed, and, also building on what she had learned of gynecology and medicine from her first husband, a provincial surgeon, she came to be recognized as a regional specialist, an expert in protracted and obstructed deliveries, a consultant to be brought in where others had failed. Schrader had mixed feelings about her fellow midwives (and doctors); some midwives she praised, some she raged against as "dreadful know-nothings," "messy bunglers," and torturers. We believe Catharina Schrader was special, perhaps unique, but in terms of learning and regulation, she was an ordinary midwife, unlicensed and unexamined, armed with what she had picked up from her husband and perhaps a few midwifery manuals, but relying for the rest on instinct, observation, manual dexterity, and experience.[15]

Attempts to resolve the disorganized state of medical practice in the Netherlands were introduced at an early stage; the nineteenth century ushered in legislation to control midwives and schools to train them. Much of this was an attempt to institute on a national basis what had been implemented in a number of Dutch towns during the last 150 years. In 1818 the first national law regulating midwives was passed (almost 100 years before regulatory legislation was achieved in England with the 1902 Midwives Act). Of great and lasting significance was the fact that midwives were regulated together with other medical practitioners, and their duties and competence vis-à-vis men-midwives and obstetric doctors outlined. The 1818 Health Act and subsequent legislation attempted to enforce uniformity, to insist on the precedence of national over local regulation and control, and to accommodate the special problem of the countryside by supplying sufficient well-trained midwives. Prior to the 1818 act, and long after it, however, rural midwives remained to all intents and purposes unregulated and beyond the law.

The 1818 act set up a system of regulation, examination, and licensing of midwives by local and provincial medical committees. It listed the fees midwives could charge and outlined their duties. Referring to three groups of obstetric practitioners—the doctor of obstetrics, the man-midwife, and the midwife—instructions for each category were drawn up. The law stipulated that a midwife had to be examined by a provincial committee of medical men before she could practice, and had to confine her practice to those births "which were natural processes or could be delivered manually, so that the midwife may never use any instruments for this purpose." She was, however, permitted to administer enemas and catheters. The midwife was instructed to call in an obstetric doctor or man-midwife in difficult or dangerous cases, and was obliged to give an annual report to the provincial committees of the complicated deliveries encountered in the course of her practice. The examination of the midwife concluded with the swearing of an oath in which she promised to maintain professional secrecy and conduct all her affairs "as a good-natured and humane midwife was supposed to do."[16]

By law, difficult births became the province of the man-midwife and obstetric doctor, but after 1818, the midwife continued to supervise the majority of normal deliveries. Later legislation of the nineteenth century was to reaffirm and reemphasize the conditions of the 1818 act, that the competence of the midwife was not to extend beyond normal physiological births, and that she was to call for help in cases beyond her competence. The second major health act of the nineteenth century, the Medical Act of 1865, restated that midwives were "only to attend such deliveries that were the work of nature or which could be executed by hand."[17]

The legislators concerned themselves primarily with defining the midwife's sphere of competence, yet they also saw the necessity of ensuring that the midwife was equipped to fulfill her role as attendant at normal births. Anxiety over the uncoordinated and unreliable system of apprenticeship training led to provision being made in the 1820s for the teaching of midwives in the "clinical schools" (*klinische scholen*). Six were established between 1824 and 1828 in towns where a hospital could provide facilities for clinical training: Amsterdam and Rotterdam, the largest and most important, Middelburg, Haarlem, Hoorn, and Alkmaar. All took midwife pupils in addition to trainee surgeons, pharmacists, and men-midwives. Admission to the schools for midwife training was restricted to women between twenty and thirty who were healthy and sturdy, literate, and of "irreproachable character." Some of the pupils were sent by local authorities for a fee of twenty guilders a year; others were admitted on a private basis. The clinical schools had many inadequacies; though the advantages of book learning were used to justify the utility of the schools over the old apprenticeship system, theoretical training was weak. Far more serious, despite the low cost of training, was the fact that the schools failed to attract midwife pupils. Between 1824 and 1867, an average of only eight women graduated from the six clinical schools each year. By 1850, of the 811 licensed midwives in the Netherlands, less than one-third had passed through the school system.

In 1861 the first state school for midwives (*Rijkskweekschool voor Vroedvrouwen*) was set up in Amsterdam, after legislation of 1860 had reaffirmed the problems of a shortage of school-trained midwives, especially in the countryside. The Amsterdam school, which taught only midwives and was intended to give a more substantial and systematic grounding in both clinical and theoretical midwifery, was followed by a second school in Rotterdam in 1882, and in 1913 a Roman Catholic school was opened in Heerlen to improve standards in the poor, rural south. In 1865 the provincial medical committees were dissolved, and a state commission took over responsibility for the examination of midwives.

Training in the state schools for midwives was free, but graduates from the schools were obliged, following the completion of the course, to practice for a number of years as midwives to the poor. There was a maximum number of pupils admitted each year; in Amsterdam twenty-six and in Rotterdam thirty-two. Each province of the Netherlands could send two women for training each year at no cost, the selection of candidates resting with provincial inspectors of public health. Private pupils were also admitted. Those admitted to the course had to be between twenty and thirty-five, preferably unmarried women or widows, and as far as possible, respectable citizens gifted with the knowledge and reason needed for thorough scientific training. The course lasted for two years, during which time the pupils boarded in the schools under the supervision of a "midwife-mistress." Training covered general anatomy and physiology, special knowledge of the female parts, the care of infants and sick women, and both theoretical and practical midwifery. Student midwives attended at deliveries in the associated clinics.

Between 1861 and 1900, the total number of pupils trained at the Amsterdam state school was 1,143 (an average of twenty-nine a year); in Rotterdam between 1882 and 1900, 628 (or thirty-five a year), which represented a major increase in the numbers passing through the six clinical schools. Although around 80 percent of those trained in the clinical schools passed the final examination, less than half of the women educated in the state schools graduated at the end of the course. Training in the state schools was recognized as being of a high standard, with a larger theoretical component than the clinical schools, but, initially, the general education of entrants was poor, hence the struggle to pass examinations. To help remedy this, a teacher who also functioned as matron and supervisor of the pupils was appointed to teach the "three Rs." In 1902 an entrance examination was instituted, and in the early decades of the twentieth century, the educational level of entrants improved (reflecting increased opportunities for secondary education for girls) to match the rigorous course requirements.[18]

COMPETITION AND CONFLICT IN THE NINETEENTH CENTURY

At the same time as the midwife was being increasingly regulated, her work defined, and her education supervised, another process, the rise of obstetricians, was taking place. Towards the close of the nineteenth century, this group was becoming increasingly involved in the birthing process. We should be wary, however, of taking the Anglo-American situation, with its associated "conflict models," as typifying what occurred in the Netherlands. The Dutch situation was much more complex; the division of tasks within midwifery, partly a result of early legislation in the Netherlands, was very different from the English or American division. While the role of the midwife narrowed during the nineteenth century—her attendance at complicated births and practice of gynecology, more common in earlier centuries, were curtailed—the midwife was not pushed out of practice in the Netherlands, though she did move increasingly into the position of attendant at normal births. While an appreciation of the shifting balance between the midwife and male obstetric practitioners is crucial to understanding the development of Dutch obstetric services and the midwife's place within these services, the claims of different groups of medical men to the right to practice obstetrics are also important.[19]

Up until the nineteenth century, the evidence suggests that medical practitioners were more concerned with regulating midwives than striving to replace them.[20] Most towns had only a small number of men-midwives, smaller centers had none, and doctors were generally only present in the birthing chamber to assist in obstructed deliveries, in cases of placenta previa, multiple births, or obstetric emergencies. The task of delivering a dead infant, or very rarely performing a Caesarean section, fell to the man-midwife or obstetric doctor. Though there was rhetoric against midwives, who were criticized for everything from a lack of skill to an absence of social graces, there was no determined effort to put them out of business. Jacob Denys, the municipal man-midwife for Leiden, railed against the midwife early in the eighteenth century: "No art is practiced in a more slovenly, reckless, and stupid way" than obstetrics by midwives. Yet he was talking about the poorly trained, the unlicensed, and both Denys and his successor, Cornelius Terne, believed the solution to lie in instruction, separating the wheat from the chaff, the ignorant, uneducated midwife from those who had followed their lessons and sworn an oath of practice. Emphasis was on reform, not replacement. Midwives were essential, all the better if they were well trained and a close eye was kept on their activities.[21]

In the nineteenth century, as in other nations, the attitude of doctors towards the practice of obstetrics was ambiguous. Many saw it as uninteresting, low status, or unremunerative, but others saw it as an important component of their work and a means of obtaining entry to better-paid practice, the oft-cited "foot in the door" to middle-class family practice. Jelle Banga, who practiced medicine and midwifery in Franeker in the northern province of Friesland between 1806 and 1873, obtained his license as man-midwife from the provincial committee in Leeuwarden in 1810, and thereafter built up an impressive obstetric practice, attending 1,100 deliveries between 1806 and 1867 (including seventeen "illegally" before taking his examination in midwifery). In 1818 Banga, together with all his man-midwife and obstetric doctor colleagues, was regulated under the Health Act, but this act regarded these two groups as obstetric specialists, not birth attendants in normal cases. Emphasizing the competence of men-midwives in obstetric emergencies, the 1818 act listed seven instruments that the man-midwife should have at his fingertips, including several types of obstetric forceps and levers.[22]

An act of 1838 revoking the ban on combined practice proved to be a critical turning point. Although survival as an obstetric doctor alone was not feasible before 1838 (there were only twenty-eight obstetric doctors in the Netherlands in 1820), after 1838, it became possible to couple obstetrics with other branches of practice (this had previously only been possible for provincial practitioners such as Banga). The number of doctors with combined qualifications, both medical and obstetric degrees, greatly increased. By 1840 there were 268 obstetric doctors, 32 percent holding both medical and obstetric degrees. The number of men-midwives more than doubled between 1820 and 1840 to 1,100. Up to the 1860s, the number of obstetric doctors and men-midwives continued to rise, and without doubt, they did not survive on obstetric emergencies alone. Although midwives seemed to be holding their own (there were 819 midwives in 1820 and 811 in 1850, despite a drop to 725 in 1860), the ratio of midwives to the general population shows continual decline from 1820 to the close of the century (see Tables 1 and 2).

In the 1860s, a new figure moved into the picture, the general practitioner (*arts*, pl. *artsen*), a creation of the Medical Act of 1865. These doctors were entitled to practice all branches of medicine, including midwifery. The categories of man-midwife and obstetric doctor were of decreasing relevance from 1865 onwards—those qualified continued to practice, but their numbers

Table 1
Obstetric Practitioners in the Netherlands, 1820–1895

Date	population	midwives	medical doctors	obstetric doctors	percentage of med. & obstet. doct.	surgeons	men-mid-wives	general practitioners
c.1820	2,109,069	819	637	28	4.4	1081	540	—
c.1840	2,705,620	811	841	268	31.9	1453	1102	—
1855	3,183,003	837	1022	457	44.7	1422	1268	—
1866	3,444,328	692*	990	586	59.2	1639	1302	8
1875	3,769,111	767	875	?	?	1010	?	132
1885	4,262,054	764	563	?	?	622	?	556
1895	4,807,776	830	384	?	?	408	?	1009

Table 2
Ratios of Obstetric Practitioners to the General Population

	midwives	men-midwives	obstetric doctors	general practitioners	men-midwives & obstet. doc.
c.1820	1:2575	1:3906	1:75324	—	1:3713
c.1840	1:3336	1:1455	1:10094	—	1:1974
1855	1:3803	1:2510	1:6701	—	1:1824
1866	1:4977*	1:2645	1:5878	1:430541	1:1824
1875	1:4914	—	—	1:28553	?
1885	1:5579	—	—	1:7666	?
1895	1:5793	—	—	1:4765	?

* All medical personnel were instructed to re-register under the medical law of 1865. The fact that many midwives chose not to re-register may explain the low figure for 1866. Even after this date, however, the ratio of midwives to the general population continued to decline.

Sources: Arntzenius, D.J.A., "Statistieke opgaven omtrent de geneeskundige bevolkingin Nederland," *Bijdrager tot de Gereeskundige Staatsregeling* 3 (1845), pp.25-53; Provincial and state medical registers. Table 1a is based on Van Lieburg and Marland, "Midwife regulation," table 3, p.302.

steadily diminished. If we wish to pinpoint the midwife's main source of competition after 1865, then it is to the general practitioner that we must turn. Between 1875 and 1895, the number of general practitioners increased almost eightfold from 132 to over 1,000. The term "general" covered not only their medical tasks, but their obstetric work as well, and they included attendance at normal deliveries in their practices. For many, such as Banga in Friesland, midwifery was not merely a sideline, but a substantial part of their practice. By 1906, 59 percent of babies born in the Netherlands were delivered by midwives, and 36 percent by medical men, mainly general practitioners.[23] Between March 1, 1908, and December 31, 1920, Herman Folmer, a general practitioner practicing in the small community of Driewegen in Zeeland, attended a total of 1,247 deliveries (an average of almost 100 a year).[24] An account of the breakdown of obstetric work for the year 1924 in the Netherlands claimed that all 2,490 general practitioners were attending births. Most were present at fewer than sixty per year (63 percent), but a significant number attended between sixty and 150 (15 percent) (see Table 3).[25]

In the Netherlands, by the turn of the twentieth century, the urban/rural divide was still of little significance, with a low level of industrialization and few major cities, yet there were still noticeable regional differences in obstetric care. In the densely populated and urbanized province of South Holland, out of a total of 41,654 births in 1906, 63 percent were midwife attended,

Table 3
Deliveries Attended by General Practitioners and Midwives in the Netherlands, 1924

general practitioners	deliveries/year	midwives	deliveries/year
1,559	1 - 30	340	1 - 50
518	31 - 60	236	50 - 100
280	61 - 100	178	101 - 150
99	101 - 150	100	150 - 200
34	over 150	116	over 200
2,490		972	

Source: Van der Hoeven, P.C.T., "Wanneer Moet de Zwangere in de Cliniek Bevallen?" *NTG 72* :II (1928), p.3978.

and 37 percent were attended by doctors. Meanwhile, in less populous North Holland, the proportions were 74 percent and 26 percent, respectively, for midwife- and doctor-attended deliveries out of a total of almost 29,397 confinements. In rural and Catholic North Brabant, however, the division was more equal between general practitioners and midwives; the former attended 40 percent of the 20,199 births, and midwives 47 percent. Some 2,615 women, almost 13 percent, gave birth in North Brabant without the assistance of either a midwife or doctor.[26]

The other source of potential competition for the midwife was the specialist obstetrician. However, as Anja Hiddinga has shown, the institutional basis of Dutch obstetrics, particularly the poor facilities for clinical research, militated against the development of obstetric research during the nineteenth century.[27] Academic training in obstetrics expanded during the century, but very slowly. In 1848 Abraham Simon Thomas (1820–86) was appointed extraordinary professor of obstetrics at the University of Leiden, but elsewhere chairs of surgery and obstetrics were combined. It was only in the 1860s that separate professorships were created at the universities of Amsterdam, Groningen, and Utrecht. Obstetrics and gynecology were included in the increase in specialist activities towards the close of the nineteenth century. The Dutch Association of Gynecologists (*Nederlandse Gynaecologische Vereniging, NGV*) was established in 1887 by a small group of Amsterdam surgeons, who two years later initiated the *Dutch Journal of Gynecology and Obstetrics* (*Nederlands Tijdschrift voor Verloskunde en Gynaecologie*). The association, however, not only had small beginnings, but it remained small, with only eighteen members by 1919, and eighty-eight by 1938. Its meetings, which were recorded in the journal, were cozy affairs with the flavor of small-town medical society gatherings. This small number of specialists was too insignificant to challenge midwives and confined their practices to specialized clinic work. The nonexpansionalist attitude and closely defined boundaries of the obstetricians, combined with the low level of institutional midwifery (by the end of the century the Amsterdam University Clinic, the largest maternity clinic in the Netherlands, was handling only around 500 deliveries a year), left normal births in the hands of the midwife and general practitioner.

THE "MIDWIFE DEBATE" AT THE TURN OF THE TWENTIETH CENTURY

Although the midwife's position as attendant at normal births had been laid down in legislation from early in the nineteenth century, with the rising involvement of the general practitioner in midwifery after the 1860s, the late nineteenth century was a period of great change, a time of challenge to the midwife. It was in this climate that the reports on the status and future of the midwife were made in 1897 and 1911. Significantly, it was the Dutch Society for the Promotion of Medicine (*Nederlandsche Maatschappij tot Bevordering der Geneeskunst*), the medical society that served as a platform for general practitioners, that initiated the reports. The aim of the reports was to assess the standard of midwife practice and to propose ways of improving their status and incomes, but the compilers of the reports, often interested parties with obstetric practices, must have had mixed motives in making their evaluations.[28]

In terms of educating and licensing, it could be expected that by this time some kind of uniformity among midwives would have been reached, but this was not the case. There was not just one group of midwives but several, with varied levels of education ranging from the young women being turned out by the two state schools, a group who had acquired their diplomas before 1865, to those lacking all formal training and working without authorization, though not necessarily lacking in skill. An impasse had been reached: it would be a matter of time before all midwives filtered through the school system and before something like uniform standards were reached. In the meantime, great concern was expressed, chiefly by medical practitioners, about midwifery practice, particularly the unqualified rural midwife, a persistent figure who was still very active in delivering babies outside the main population centers until the 1930s.

In the southern Catholic province of North Brabant, there was a desperate shortage of trained midwives up to World War II; villages were often without either a midwife or a doctor, and very few women left the province to attend one of the state schools. In 1869, there was only one midwife for every 11,591 inhabitants in North Brabant, compared with one for 4,972 nationally. By 1935, the difference had narrowed considerably—with one midwife per 10,121 inhabitants in North Brabant, and one to every 8,524 nationally (also a revealing figure)—but the gap between need and help often had to be filled by neighbors, mothers, and unqualified "*bakers*" (dry nurses who helped mothers following confinement).[29] In 1869 only one out of the thirty-seven midwives practicing in North Brabant had attended one of the state schools (3 percent), by 1899 this had increased to 55 percent, and in 1920 to 77 percent, but still one-quarter of working midwives lacked an official education.[30] Concern about the standard of midwife practice was closely related to efforts to reduce infant mortality, which was partly attributed to poor obstetric services.

There were local black spots, chiefly the poor rural areas in the south of the country, where both infant and maternal mortality remained high, regions that lacked qualified midwives and supporting maternity services. For the years 1901–05, the national infant death rate was 136 per 1,000, but this hid great regional variations: 136 per 1,000 in the urbanized province of South Holland, ninety-two and 109 in the northern rural provinces of Friesland and Groningen, and 173 and 183 in the southern rural and predominantly Catholic provinces of Limburg and North Brabant.[31] Infant death rates remained above the national average in North Brabant well into the 1930s. One general practitioner writing on the region maintained in 1922 that the "modern midwife" who had learned how to care for newborn babies hygienically would be a vital figure in reducing infant mortality.[32] Areas such as North Brabant were specially targeted by infant welfare workers, but because of poverty, isolation, religious belief, and low levels of education, they were also the areas that reformers found most difficult to reach.

The reports of 1897 and 1911 were largely intended to resolve the problem of low standards in the countryside, yet the data they provide related little to unqualified practice. Most of the information centered on licensed midwives, the visible strata who had contact in the course of their practices with the medical practitioners compiling the evidence. In 1897, 354 midwives were included in the sample based on doctors' replies; 480 doctor respondents gave information in 1911. Although significant portions of the licensed midwife population were included, the reports were far from representative. The reports were also concerned with good obstetric standards from the point of view of medical practitioners. Data on the midwives' knowledge of asepsis and a variety of medical techniques were collected, yet no survey was made of the number of births carried out by midwives each year, a reflection of the compilers' interest in formal training and medical competence above practical skill and experience. Emphasis was also placed on the necessity of summoning a doctor in good time in difficult cases. On this point, both reports were fairly positive, stating that around 80 percent of midwives called for assistance in good time.

What then were the conclusions of the reports? Some 60 percent of the medical practitioners responding to the 1897 questionnaire described the skills and theoretical knowledge of midwives as "good" or "very good," but this still left some 40 percent of midwives who were considered average or bad. Similarly, 60 percent were considered proficient in antiseptic techniques.[33] The report also analyzed the incomes of midwives in great detail. Generally, these were made up of payments by a town or region for attendance on the poor, which could take the form of a fixed payment or fee per case, and the fees of private patients, although occasionally medical men also paid midwives a fixed amount for attendance at deliveries in a system of "farming out" cases. The incomes of midwives, whatever their source, were subject to great variation. Before 1865, the fees of midwives were set in accordance with tariffs drawn up for all medical practitioners, guaranteeing some uniformity. After 1865 they fell outside of this scale of tariffs, midwives entering in effect the "free market." The fees paid to town midwives, for example, bore little relation to the number of deliveries attended, and ranged from the 150 guilders paid by the Amsterdam town council for attendance at more than 100 deliveries a year (less than 1.50 guilders per case), to the 400 guilders paid to the town midwife of 's-Hertogenbosch in the east of the Netherlands for an unknown but presumably much smaller number of deliveries. Private fees also varied greatly, according to the wealth of the town or region, and the availability of obstetric assistance. The report calculated that the fees paid by laborers and lower middle-class groups to midwives averaged 2.50 to 5 guilders, but the range could be much wider in either direction. In the province of North Holland, the usual fee was 4 to 5 guilders for a normal birth; in poverty-stricken North Brabant, 2.50 to 4 guilders was the average, but fees as low as 50 cents were also recorded. Yearly incomes were also subject to great variation. These could be less than 300 guilders or more than 800, but an average for the country as a whole was given as 500 to 600 guilders a year, an increase on the 200 to 300 guilders cited as an average in the early nineteenth century.[34]

The report found that doctors often tried to undercut midwives by charging low fees, leaving the midwife with only the very poor as clients. It was recommended that medical men should offer more support to midwives and avoid direct competition with them, enabling them to maintain their practices. Without this support, no patients would be left for the midwife to attend. Yet, in practical terms, little was achieved. The 1911 report declared that unfair competition by general practitioners remained a major problem for the midwife. Few of the recommendations of the 1897 respondents—for stricter admissions procedures to the state schools, compulsory use of aseptic techniques, the establishment of retraining courses, for eliminating unqualified midwives, or for raising fees and the salaries of town midwives—were acted on, and all were reiterated in 1911. One of the few concrete spin-offs of the report was the founding of a journal for midwives in 1897, the *Journal of Practical Midwifery* (*Maandblad voor Praktische Verloskunde*, and from 1899, *Tijdschrift voor Praktische Verloskunde*), by two members of the committee of inquiry, Meinart Niemeyer (1861–1934), a provincial general practitioner, and G. C. Nijhoff (1857–1932), professor of obstetrics and gynecology in Groningen. The *Tijdschrift voor Praktische Verloskunde* functioned as a platform for Dutch midwives. It included articles on obstetric practices, maternity services, and information on the position of midwives in the Netherlands and abroad. Yet doctors had editorial control, and the opinions expressed by the midwife authors were often challenged by the editors. Also in

1897, the Dutch Society of Midwives (*Bond van Nederlandse Vroedvrouwen*) was founded, which by 1898 had around 300 members.

The perceived lack of improvement in the quality of midwives' practices resulted in the drawing up of another, substantially more detailed, report in 1911. This report again offered evidence of male medical practitioners' perceptions of midwives, though this time the report was prepared jointly by the Dutch Society for the Promotion of Medicine and the Dutch Association of Gynecologists. The main elements of the questionnaire are shown in Table 4. With regard to midwives' knowledge and skills, the respondents were positive, much more so than in the 1897 report. More than 80 percent described the obstetric skills of midwives as good or satisfactory; over 70 percent claimed that midwives were familiar with aseptic techniques. However, 61 percent of the respondents concluded that midwives did not conduct proper examinations of pregnant women, and some 63 percent claimed that urine examinations were not made. There were few specific complaints: out of 480 responses, nine cases were cited in which midwives were considered to have overstepped their duties; twenty-eight midwives, it was claimed, attended too many deliveries; and there were fifty-eight vague charges of indifference, conceit, indolence, and untrustworthiness. Although most of the respondents believed that a refresher course for midwives would be of value, 84 percent also believed that their competence should not be extended.[35] It is perhaps this

Table 4

Evaluation of Midwives by General Practitioners in the Netherlands, 1911

	good	satisfactory	moderate	bad	no answer	general opinion
general knowledge	59	178	112	84	47	+
theoretical knowledge	92	214	61	66	47	+
midwifery skills	197	199	17	23	45	+

Did midwives' practice include:	yes	no	no answer	general opinion
pregnancy examination	131	291	58	-
urine examination	141	303	46	-
correct diagnosis	377	64	39	+
calling timely assistance	380	70	30	+
supervision of nursing	216	218	46	=
use of aseptic techniques	342	107	31	+
birth control advice*	63	381	36	-
refresher course necessary	291	103	86	-
extension of competence recommended	53	402	25	-

+ generally positive responses
- generally negative responses
= responses evenly divided

* The low figure for dispensing birth control advice by midwives was largely the result of respondents' equating the birth control question with assistance in abortions.

Number of doctors responding: 480

Source: "Report," 1911, pp.1130-31. Table is based on Van Lieburg and Marland, "Midwife regulation," table 6, p.313.

last response that gives us the most insight into the status quo between mid-wives and doctors in the Netherlands in 1911.

What was the response to the reports of 1897 and 1911? The reaction of the medical profession to both reports was remarkably muted, perhaps indicative of the status of the reports, which informed on the situation and proposed small amendments rather than any fundamental attempt to reform obstetric services. The medical journals made little mention of the reports, though it was significant that one of the midwife's most vehement opponents, A. Geyl (1853–1914), surgeon, gynecologist, and would-be medical historian, chose the years 1897 and 1911 to publish a series of articles attacking mid-wives in the *Medisch Weekblad.* Geyl discussed the status of midwives in the fifteenth to eighteenth centuries, concluding that they were generally un-skilled, careless, brutal, and lacking integrity and a sense of duty, but it is clear that his articles, coinciding closely with the publication of the reports, were intended to reflect on the status of the midwife at the turn of the twentieth century.[36]

Also appearing in 1911 was Catharine van Tussenbroek's classic work, *De Ontwikkeling der Aseptische Verloskunde* (The Development of Aseptic Obstetrics), which was more positive about the history of the midwife and her contribution to Dutch obstetric services. Praising the midwife for her high standards and low rates of childbed fever, Van Tussenbroek expressed anxiety about the declining ratio of midwives to the population, which had fallen off from eighteen midwives to every 100,000 population in 1891 (807 midwives) to fifteen per 100,000 in 1908 (882 midwives). Van Tussenbroek, the second woman to qualify in medicine in the Netherlands and a highly respected gynecologist, was a member of the committee responsible for organizing the 1911 report. Nevertheless, she was highly critical of the findings of both the 1897 and 1911 reports. She was bitterly opposed to the suggestions that by insisting on an improvement in the antiseptic and hygienic standards of midwives, their status would be improved, and that by reducing the competition of general practitioners, midwives' salaries be raised to a reasonable level and their positions would become tolerable. "A tolerable position! there lies the core of the whole midwife question. The midwife, with her carefully organized, two-year training—an example to foreign countries—on top of her exhausting, because heavily responsible, position, she must face financial uncertainty, together with a poor future."[37]

One crucial difference between the reports of 1897 and 1911 was that mid-wives were given the right to reply in 1911. A questionnaire was forwarded to 896 licensed midwives, and some 424 (47.3 percent) responded. The mid-wives, however, were asked a rather different set of questions to those put to the doctor respondents, questions that largely dealt with the midwives' train-ing and their satisfaction with the course offered. Many believed changes were necessary—some 40 percent concluded that more practical experience would be beneficial, 29 percent more nursing, but only 17 percent thought that the course should have a larger theoretical content. A surprising 79 percent believed that retraining would be beneficial. The midwife respondents had very different answers to questions concerning their standard of practice from the doctors who had completed the questionnaire. About 76 percent of midwives claimed that they carried out adequate prenatal examinations (compared with 27 percent of doctor respondents); 40 percent that they made urine examinations (compared with 29 percent); and, most significantly, some 280 midwives (67 percent) believed that their competence should be extended (compared with 11 percent). Midwives were particularly keen to obtain the right to use forceps (40 percent), to stitch the perineum, and to give injections.[38]

What was in effect a demand by midwives for the authorization to carry out instrumental deliveries is particularly significant—it was also campaigned for in the *Tijdschrift voor Praktische Verloskunde.* The demand raises interesting questions about the role of the midwife as attendant and advocate of normal births. Midwives believed that an extension of their competence would not only improve their professional status, but would also be in the interests of mothers and babies. Very few midwives saw unqualified practitioners as a serious challenge, but one-third believed that the competition from general practitioners undermined their practices. As a Zeeland midwife commented, the ups and downs of a midwife depend largely on the relationship between her and the general practitioner functioning above her.[39] More radical views were expressed by midwives in the *Tijdschrift voor Praktische Verloskunde.* In a series of twelve articles, J. A. van den Brink, one of the journal's editors, took upon himself the task of summarizing the findings of the 1911 report, but his summary came far from satisfying all the journal's midwife readership. One anonymous writer (identified by the editors as Mej. K. Sybrandy-Miedema, a regular correspondent), argued that it was time to call a halt to all the "nonsensical" talk about the position of the midwife. "It is more than time that the Dutch woman is brought again to realize that pregnancy, birth, and lying-in are normal affairs. We midwives must grasp firmly to the idea that *all* births are ours, nothing less."[40]

The recommendations of the reports of 1897 and 1911 rested largely on the premise that normal births were the responsibility of the midwife, and abnormal ones the responsibility of the general practitioner or obstetrician. Admission to the midwife schools and training should be tightened up, and refresher courses organized, but an extension of midwives' competence was "not desirable" and would be against the interests of patients. Doctors were to stop behaving badly towards midwives in their area, which would diminish complaints on both sides.[41]

Increasingly during the nineteenth century doctors took it upon themselves to judge the midwife, her competence, how she should be trained, and what she should be doing. Though many doctors were very positive about the midwife's role in obstetric services—"I would rather that my wife was delivered by a good midwife, than by 80 percent of the general practitioners"[42]—the doctors set themselves up in a judgmental and superior position to midwives. Their attitude was somewhat patronizing, offering condolences for the midwife's partial loss of authority in the form of promises of improved salaries and better working relationships. Midwives in the Netherlands seem to have offered little resistance to this process. They were relatively late to organize, and, compared to England and the United States, were less vocal, less active in the women's movement, and less able to muster the support of pressure groups of women doctors.[43]

Although in other nations, especially the United States, some sections of the medical profession (in the end, those who achieved their aims) wished to squeeze the midwife out of independent practice, in the Netherlands, doctors settled for a division of labor, with the midwife sharing responsibility with the general practitioner for normal home (and later short-stay hospital) deliveries. Although the midwife lost out in many ways during the nineteenth century, as increased regulation diminished her involvement in complicated deliveries and closed off any hope of practicing gynecology, in some sense, this was inevitable. In the face of advances in medical technology and institutionalization, the midwife was fated to be restricted if she were to continue to be the usual attendant at normal births. The Dutch midwife retained a high level of autonomy, and a workable compromise was reached, which was largely responsible for the independence of the Dutch midwife and the high level of home births today.

The legislation of the nineteenth century, which made the midwife responsible for normal births but nothing more, spelled out the situation not only for the midwife, but also for the obstetrician and general practitioner. Also, though the midwife lost some ground and some potential, so did male obstetric practitioners. The slow development of institutional obstetrics denied the obstetrician an environment in which he could deliver many women. The founding of midwife schools, which gradually enabled the midwife to achieve the standards believed to be necessary for good practice, ensured that what had been given could not be taken away. A good training was the midwife's insurance and bulwark against competition. By the early twentieth century, a status quo had been reached, not always a comfortable or stable status quo, but nevertheless one that assured the position of midwives as "the guardians of normal birth."[44]

NOTES

Several sections of this chapter were based on Van Lieburg, M. J., and Hilary Marland, "Midwife regulation, education, and practice in the Netherlands during the nineteenth century," *Medical History* 33 (1989): 296–317. I would like to thank Lara Marks and Irvine Loudon for commenting upon an earlier version of this article.

1. *See* Jordan, Brigitte, *Birth in Four Cultures: A Crosscultural Investigation of*

Childbirth in Yucatan, Holland, Sweden and the United States (Montreal: Eden Press Women's Publications, 1978); World Health Organization, *Having a Baby in Europe* (Public Health in Europe 26, Copenhagen, 1985); and the chapters by Eva Abraham-Van der Mark and L. H. Lumey in this volume.

2. Sullivan, Deborah A., and Rose Weitz, *Labor Pains: Modern Midwives and Home Birth* (New Haven: Yale University Press, 1988): 36, 71; DeVries, Raymond G., *Regulating Birth: Midwives, Medicine and the Law* (Philadelphia: Temple University Press, 1985): 50. Figures given for Caesarean section in 1981 are 3.6 percent for the Netherlands, 7.3 percent for England, 12.7 percent for West Germany, and 15.4 percent for Greece (the highest of the thirteen countries cited). *See* Phaff, J.M.L., "De Nederlandse verloskunde in Europees perspectief," in *Voortgang en Visie: 25 Jaar Verloskunde en Gynaecologie*, Treffers, P. E., et al. (eds.) (Utrecht: Scheltema & Holkema, 1983): 6.

3. Tew, Marjorie, *Safer Childbirth? A Critical History of Maternity Care* (London: Chapman and Hall, 1990), 270.

4. Van Lieburg, M. J., and Hilary Marland, "Midwife regulation, education, and practice in the Netherlands during the nineteenth century," *Medical History* 33 (1989): 296–317; van Gelder, Floor, "Is Dat nu Typies Vrouwenwerk? De Maatschappelijke Positie van Vroedvrouwen," *Tijdschrift voor Vrouwenstudies* 3 (1982): 5–33; van der Borg, Els, "Wijze Volksvrouwen. Beroepsvorming van Vroedvrouwen in Nederland tot 1865," *Focaal. Tijdschrift voor Antropologie* 14 (1990): 13–34.

5. For the United States, for example, *see* Leavitt, Judith Walzer, *Brought to Bed: Childbearing in America, 1750–1950* (New York: Oxford University Press, 1986): chapter 7.

6. By the 1880s, there were only four lying-in clinics in the Netherlands. These were connected to the medical faculties at Amsterdam, Utrecht, Leiden, and Groningen. A small number of deliveries were also carried out in clinics attached to the two state midwife schools in Amsterdam and Rotterdam, but by the close of the century, hospital births probably did not exceed 1,000 per year. Van Lieburg and Marland, "Midwife regulation," p. 314.

In 1960 only 26 percent of the 242,407 deliveries in the Netherlands took place in a hospital; the other 74 percent were home births. Meanwhile, in the United States in 1957, 96 percent of births took place in a hospital. By 1965 the proportion of home births in the Netherlands had been reduced to 68.6 percent, and by 1975 to 44.4 percent. In 1983, 35.1 percent of the babies delivered in the Netherlands were born at home. In 1910, about 60 percent of all births in the Netherlands were attended by midwives. This percentage gradually fell to 48 percent in 1940, 41 percent in 1950, 37 percent in 1960, and 36.7 percent in 1970. By 1977 there had been a small increase in the percentage of babies delivered by midwives. Out of the 175,000 babies born in the Netherlands, 37.8 percent were delivered by midwives (an average of eighty-four per midwife per year, and a total of 66,000 deliveries). By 1983 the proportion of births attended by midwives had again risen; 57.7 percent of the 171,000 deliveries in 1983 were attended by doctors, and 41.6 percent by midwives. Snapper, I., "Midwifery, past and present," *Bulletin of the New York Academy of Medicine* 39 (1963): 526; Klinkert, J. J., *Verloskundigen en Artsen Verleden en Heden van Enkele Professionele Beroepen in de Gezondheidzorg* (Alphen aan den Rijn/Brussels:

Stafleu, 1980): 66, 72; Centraal Bureau voor de Statistiek, *1899–1979 Tachtig Jaren Statistiek in Tijdreeksen* (The Hague: Staatsuitgeverij, 1979); *Statistisch Zakboek 1985.*

7. Darlington, Thomas, "The present status of the midwife," *American Journal of Obstetrics and Gynecology* 63 (1911): 870. *See* also Litoff, Judy Barrett, "Forgotten women: American midwives at the turn of the twentieth century," *Historian* 40 (1978): 235–351.

8. Kobrin, Frances E., "The American midwife controversy: a crisis of profession-alization," *Bulletin of the History of Medicine* 40 (1966): 351.

9. Towler, Jean, and Joan Bramall, *Midwives in History and Society* (London: Croom Helm, 1986): chapter 8; Carter, Jenny, and Thérèse Duriez, *With Child: Birth Through the Ages* (Edinburgh: Mainstream Publishing, 1986).

10. Kobrin, "The American midwife controversy"; Litoff, Judy Barrett, *The American Midwife Debate: A Sourcebook on Its Modern Origins* (Westport, CT: Greenwood Press, 1986); Devitt, Neal, "The statistical case for elimination of the midwife: fact versus prejudice, 1890–1935," *Women and Health* 4 (1979): 81–96, 169–186.

11. Donnison, Jean, *Midwives and Medical Men: A History of Inter-Professional Rivalries and Women's Rights* (New York: Schocken, 1977).

12. "Dutch Society for the Promotion of Medicine: Report of the Committee to In-vestigate the Means by Which Medical Men Can Improve the Standard and Status of Midwives in the Netherlands" (*Nederlandsche Maatschappij tot Bevordering der Geneeskunst. Rapport der Commissie ter Onderzoek naar de Wijze Waarop door Geneeskundigen, Verbetering Gebracht kan Worden in het Gehalte en Positie der Vroedvrouwen in Nederland*), March (1897), in *Nederlands Tijdschrift voor Geneeskunde* 33:I (1897): 610–628; "Report of the Commission Selected by the Dutch Society for the Promotion of Medicine and the Dutch Association of Gynecolo-gists on Midwifery Practice in the Netherlands" (*Nederlandsche Maatschappij tot Bevordering der Geneeskunst. Rapport der Commissie in Zake het Vroedv-rouwenvraagstuk hier te Lande, Benoemd door het Hoofdbestuur der Nederlandsche Maatschappij tot Bevordering der Geneeskunst in Samenwerking met het Bestuur der Nederlandsche Gynaecologische Vereeniging*) February (1911), in *Nederlands Tijdschrift voor Geneeskunde (NTG)* 55:IA (1911): 1105–1132.

13. "The guardian of normal birth" comes from Tew, *Safer Childbirth?*, p. 68.

14. For midwives during the early modern period, *see*, for example, van der Borg, Els, "Beeldvorming over Vroedvrouwen in de Noordelijke Nederlanden (1600–1900)," *Verzorging* 3 (1988): 2–17; van der Borg, H. A., *Vroedvrouwen; Beeld en Beroep Ontwikkelingen in het Vroedvrouwschap in Leider, Arnhem, s'-Hertogerbosch en Leeuwarden*, Proefschrift, University of Amsterdam (Wageningen: Wageningen Aca-demic Press, 1992): van Lieburg, M. J. and Hilary Marland, "Elisabeth en Neeltje van Putten: Twee 18e-Eeuwse Grensgangers Tussen de Beroepsvelden van Vroedvrouw en Vroedmeester," *Tijdschrift voor de Geschiedenis der Geneeskunde, Natuurwetenschappen, Wiskunde en Techniek* 12 (1989): 181–197; Marland, Hilary, "The '*burgerlijke*' midwife: The *Stadsvroedvrouw* of eighteenth-century Holland," in Marland, Hilary (ed.), *The Art of Midwifery: Early Modern Midwives in Europe* (Lon-don: Routledge, 1993), 192–213.

15. Marland, Hilary, M. J. van Lieburg, and G. J. Kloosterman, p. 68. "*Mother and Child Were Saved*": *The Memoirs (1693–1740) of the Frisian Midwife Catharina*

Schrader (Amsterdam: Rodopi, 1987). For a brief summary of Schrader's life and work, *see* Marland, Hilary, "All well for mother and child: The notebook and practice of Vrouw Catharina Schrader, 1693–1745," *Nursing Times* 83 (October 7, 1987): 49–51, and Schama, Simon, *The Embarrassment of Riches: An Interpretation of Dutch Culture in the Golden Age* (London: William Collins, 1987): 525–535. In Dutch, see also, the fuller transcription of Vrouw Schrader's notebook with introductory essays, van Lieburg, M. J. (ed.), *C. G. Schrader's Memoryboeck van de Vrouwens. Het Notitieboek van een Friese Vroedvrouw 1693–1745* (with an obstetric commentary by G. J. Kloosterman) (Amsterdam: Rodopi, 1984).

16. *Verzameling van Wetten, Besluiten en Regelementen, Betrekkelijk de Burgerlijke Geneeskundige Dienst in het Koningrijk der Nederlanden* (The Hague: J. P. Beekman, 1836): 197. For more details on nineteenth-century midwife legislation, *see* van Lieburg and Marland, "Midwife regulation."

17. Klinkert, *Verloskundigen en Artsen*, p. 40.

18. Van Lieburg, M. J., "De Rijksweekschool voor Vroedvrouwen 1882–1926," in Scholte, E., van Lieburg, M. J., and Aalbersberg, R. O., *Rijksweekschool voor Vroedvrouwen te Rotterdam* (Leidschendam: Ministerie van Volksgezondheid en Milieuhygiëne, 1982) chapter 2.

19. As Ornella Moscucci has recently shown, the situation in England was also much more complex than a simple tussle between the midwife and her male rivals. A variety of medical groups, doctors of physic, surgeons, and general practitioners, all laid claim to the authority to practice obstetrics and gynecology during the course of the nineteenth century. Towards the century's close, the struggle focused increasingly on the conflict between obstetricians and general surgeons over the right to perform abdominal surgery. Moscucci, Ornella, *The Science of Women, Gynaecology and Gender in England, 1800–1929* (Cambridge: Cambridge University Press, 1990).

20. This also seems to have been the case in the Germanys during the eighteenth century. Male accoucheurs did not muscle women out of the birthing room, but there were attempts to "reform" midwifery, to "improve" the instruction of midwives, and to "discipline" them. *See* Lindemann, Mary, "Professionals? Sisters? Rivals? Midwives in Braunschweig, 1750–1800," in Marland (ed.), *The Art of Midwifery*, pp. 176–191.

21. Denys, Jacobus, *Verhandelingen over het Ampt der Vroed-vrouwen en Vroed-meesters* (Leiden: Juriaan Wishoff, 1733), p. 1. Cited Van der Borg, "Beeldvorming over Vroedvrouwen," p. 6; Terne, Cornelius, *Lucina. Ontdekkende de Waare Oorzaken* (Leiden: C. F. Koening, 1784). See also van der Borg, Els, "Het Ontslag van de Stadsvroedmeester Cornelius Terne. Wedijverende Beroepsgroepen te Leiden in de Achttiende Eeuw," *Holland* 2 (1990): 109–120.

22. Van Lieburg, M. J., *Jelle Banga (1786–1877). Notulist van de 19de-Eeuwse Genees- en Verloskunde in een Friese Provinciestad* (Rotterdam: Erasmus Publishing, 1991), pp. 59, 61.

23. The remaining 5 percent gave birth without obstetric assistance. Catharine van Tussenbroek, *De Ontwikkeling der Aseptische Verloskunde in Nederland* (Haarlem: De Erven F. Bohn, 1911), p. 183.

24. Folmer, Herman Reinders, *Verslag van 1247 Baringen*, Proefschrift, University of Amsterdam (Goes: Oosterbaan & Le Cointre, 1923), p. 20.

25. Van der Hoeven, P.C.T., "Wanneer Moet de Zwangere in de Cliniek Bevallen?" *NTG* 72: II (1928), p. 3978.

26. Van Tussenbroek, *De Ontwikkeling der Aseptische Verloskunde*, p. 185.

27. *See* Hiddinga, Anja, "Obstetrical research in the Netherlands in the nineteenth century," *Medical History* 31 (1987): 281–305, and the chapter by Hiddinga in this volume.

28. The Dutch Society for the Promotion of Medicine was founded in 1849 by a group of young progressive doctors as the first national medical organization in the Netherlands. Its primary aim was to change the medical law of 1818 and to move towards a medical profession unified in terms of education and licensing. First dominated by medical doctors and town surgeons, support grew only slowly, and it took until 1876 before the society's membership included more than half of the profession. It was one of the forces behind the 1865 medical act, which created the general practitioner.

29. Very different from the *kraamverpleegster*, the maternity home-care assistant, trained with one of the *kruisvereenigingen* ("cross societies," private organizations set up to improve maternity and other preventive health services) or the *Nederlandsche Bond tot Bescherming van Zuigelingen* (the Dutch Confederation for the Protection of Infants, set up in 1908 by a group of pediatricians and obstetricians to coordinate work in infant welfare), and with a diploma to work as a maternity nurse. For the development of maternity and infant welfare services, *see* Marland, Hilary, "The institutionalization of motherhood: Doctors and infant welfare in the Netherlands, 1901–1930," in *Women and Children First: International Maternal and Infant Welfare, 1870–1945*, Fildes, Valerie, Lara Marks, and Hilary Marland (eds.) (London: Routledge, 1992) pp. 74–96; and the chapter by Edwin van Teijlingen in this volume.

30. Pruijt, Marga, "Roeien, Baren en in de Arbeid Zijn. Vroedvrouwen in Noord-Brabant, 1880–1960," in Maria Grever and Annemiek van der Veen (eds.), *Bij ons moeder en ons Jet. Brabantse vrouwen in de 19de en 20ste eeuw* (Zutphen: De Walburg Pers, 1989), pp. 126, 129.

31. Vandenbroeke, C., F. van Poppel, and A. M. van der Woude, "De Zuigelingen-en Kindersterfte in België en Nederland in Seculair Perspectief," *Tijdschrijft voor Gescheidenis* 94 (1981): 481. Religious practices seem to have influenced regional mortality variations, including infant deaths. In the Catholic regions of the south, shorter periods of maternal breastfeeding, the tradition of binding the breasts of young girls, and low levels of schooling were all potential influences on infant survival. *See* van Poppel, F., "Religion and health: Catholicism and regional mortality differences in nineteenth-century Netherlands," *Social History of Medicine* 5 (1992): 229–253.

32. Barentsen, P. A., "Over de Kindersterfte ten Plattenlande van Oost-Noordbrabant," *NTG* 66:IIA (1922): 610–622.

33. "Report," 1897, p. 612.

34. Ibid., pp. 615–617. In general, the salaries of nurses during this period were much lower. During the late nineteenth century, nurses in the Buitengasthuis, Amsterdam, were earning only 150 to 200 guilders per year. Van Tussenbroek, *De Ontwikkeling der Aseptische Verloskunde*, p. 94.

35. "Report," 1911, pp. 1130–1134.

36. Geyl, A., "Over de Opleiding en Maatschappelijke Positie der Vroedvrouwen

in de 17de en 18de Eeuw," *Medisch Weekblad* 4 (1897–98): 6–10, 18–26, 35–41, 53–62, 67–73, 86–90, 115–117; "Beschouwingen en Mededeelingen over Vroedvrouwen uit de 15de tot en met de 18de Eeuw," *Medisch Weekblad* 18 (1911–12): 227–231, 266–270, 279–283, 318–322, 341–345, 353–357, 368–369, 377–381, 401–406, 414–417, 425–430.

37. Van Tussenbroek, *De Ontwikkeling der Aseptische Verloskunde*, p. 215.

38. "Report," 1911, pp. 1130–1131, 1148, 1152, 1157.

39. "Report," 1911, pp. 1161–1162.

40. Vroedvrouw, Een, "De 'Klassenstrijd' in de Vroedvrouwenwereld," *Tijdschrift voor Praktische Verloskunde* 15:3 (1911): 50.

41. "Report," 1911, pp. 1180–1181.

42. Statement of an unidentified doctor. Cited in van den Brink, J. A., "Kraambedsterfte in Nederland," *Tijdschrift voor Praktische Verloskunde* 15:6 (1911): 100.

43. Donnison, *Midwives and Medical Men*; Litoff, *The American Midwife Debate*, especially chapter 5.

44. Many areas remain controversial today, for example, the low remuneration of midwives compared with general practitioners, competition with the general practitioner in rural areas, and the problems surrounding the introduction of additional technical procedures in pregnancy and birth. *See* van der Hulst, L.A.M. (ed.), *De Vroedvrouw, de Spil van de Verloskunde* (Bilthoven: Catharina Schrader Stichting, 1991).

3

Dutch Obstetric Science: Emergence, Growth, and Present Situation

Anja Hiddinga

Although the practice of midwifery in the Netherlands has been discussed extensively, there are no thorough studies of the science of Dutch midwifery: obstetrics. Given the special situation of birth practices in the Netherlands, such a lack is surprising. The absence of scholarly interest on the part of historians is especially regrettable. Because cognitive and social processes are intimately linked and they cannot be properly understood apart from one another, the special structure of Dutch practice surrounding childbirth and delivery raises intriguing questions about the research that has underpinned it. Complementing historical studies of the practice itself, historical analyses of the science of obstetrics would help us understand how the practice acquired its special character and how it has been maintained to the present day.

Dutch medical science provides an interesting comparison with German medicine, which has been extensively studied. Germany is considered the place where scientific medicine in general, and physiology and clinical medicine in particular, were first established and developed most rapidly. The Netherlands is a neighboring country with traditional close ties to Germany, and reception of the new German scientific medicine in the Netherlands, as well as the different social circumstances there, need to be understood. The focus on one particular specialty in such a historical study allows us to specify the development with sufficient precision.

It is important to investigate not only organizational aspects and institutional changes, but also changes in the ideal of medical sciences as interpreted or understood in the Netherlands. The available literature on clinical medicine in Germany will be used heuristically, and no thorough comparison

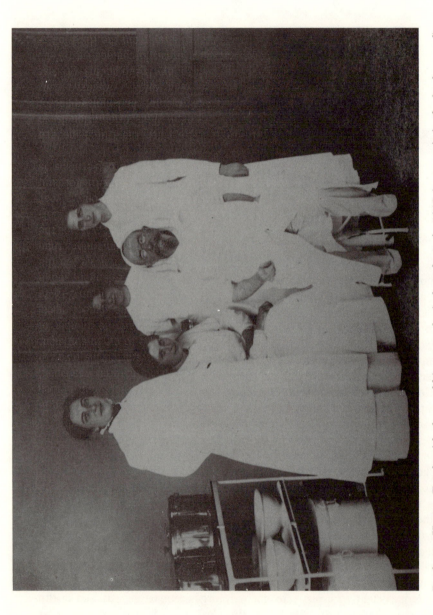

Professor Hector Treub with three of his gynecological students in 1917 (a nurse is in the background). Used by permission of Anja Hiddinga. This photograph was kindly provided by Mevr. Dr. E. J. Schaepman-van Geuns.

of the Dutch and German situation will be attempted. Such an enterprise would require more quantitative data and information about the social and political setting of science in the Netherlands than is currently available. Thus, the available knowledge about science in Germany will be used as a guide to possible explanations. Obstetrics, one of the oldest medical specialties within the biomedical sciences, provides an opportunity for studying cognitive development in relation to radical changes in the intellectual climate of nineteenth-century society.

This discussion will focus first on the organizational aspects of the emergence of medical science in the Netherlands, with special attention to the reorganization of Dutch medical legislation. We shall find a group of doctors voicing professional demands and organizing themselves to promote their ideal of clinical science. A discussion of the particular form and direction of this ideal in the Netherlands, and of the research effort it gave rise to, will be followed by a closer study of Dutch obstetrics, which failed to develop a research tradition comparable to the German model. An explanation for this leads us to examine the conditions of clinical practice in obstetrics, its institutional setting, and its intellectual context. We conclude with a look at the current situation in Dutch obstetrics in the light of its historical development.

THE REORGANIZATION OF DUTCH MEDICAL LEGISLATION

The very complicated and lengthy development of medical legislation in the Netherlands in the nineteenth century can only be broadly outlined here. Much of it needs to be understood in the context of the turbulent social and political changes that took place in Dutch society. By the end of the century, the socio-political situation in the relatively young Dutch state bore little resemblance to that at the beginning of the century.[1] Although these processes are of major importance for understanding the development of the Netherlands, they can here be sketched in only as a background against which the struggles for the legal organization of medical education and medical authority should be understood.

The first law regulating the issuing of medical licenses was passed in 1818. It reinforced the existing division between graduates (university-trained doctors with a largely theoretical education) and those trained through apprenticeship. In order to graduate, university-trained doctors were required to write a dissertation in one of three disciplines: internal medicine, obstetrics, or surgery. This gave them the right to practice in only that one area. The extent to which they could combine more than one of these practices was limited, even if they had graduated in all three.

After 1818 the nongraduate doctors (city healing-masters, country healing-masters, male and female midwives, surgeons, tooth-masters, etc.) were required to pass an examination before a local departmental or provincial committee composed of graduate doctors. The issuing of licenses to nongraduate doctors differed widely, but the most evident distinction was between country and city doctors. Usually the nongraduate doctors acquired the skills and knowledge needed to pass the examination via an apprenticeship in an existing practice or by attending a private school. Clinical schools were established by the state in 1823 in order to improve the clinical training of the nongraduate doctors. In 1830, however, the requirement of school attendance prior to examinations was dropped again. Following this change, anyone could attempt to pass the examinations, however or wherever he might have acquired his knowledge and skill.

The laws of 1818 and 1823 are the two most important ones regulating medical practice in the first half of the century: they were subsequently altered slightly and extended. The measures proposed, however, could hardly be implemented because of the lack of proper institutions to enforce them and the declining interest of committee members. Moreover, adherence to the laws could not be monitored sufficiently.

In general, this period of Dutch history is characterized by historians as one of uncertainty about the future of the new state. When the French occupation ceased in 1813, the Netherlands became "the stagnating and placid society of the 1820s."[2] The revolution of the Belgians in 1830 and their subsequent separation from the Netherlands created more political instability, but at the same time made room for a sense of national identity. "Only after 1840 did the Dutch, under constantly deteriorating economic circumstances, start trying to develop their political system."[3] Repeated attempts on the part of the government to bring order into the variety of licenses available in the medical occupations during the first decades of the nineteenth century have to be seen in this light.

Medical groups, faced with a sequence of changes in laws regulating education and licensing, were unable to develop a common perspective. Because of the limitations on their practice, the graduate *doctores medicinae, doctores artis obstetricae,* and *doctores chirurgiae* were at a disadvantage compared to the nongraduate doctors, even though the nongraduates had to call on them for help in special cases (mainly operations). Given the considerable growth in the number of doctors, especially nongraduates, this situation led in the 1830s and 1840s to a growing polarization and competition between graduates and nongraduates. Finally, in order to regulate the medical profession, a state committee without representatives of the nongraduate doctors was installed in 1848 to advise the government.

The graduate doctors did not constitute a homogeneous group. Conservative as well as progressive sentiments were expressed, but the proponents of the more modern view were the most outspoken. We shall examine later the content and character of these ideas. Three professors on the committee belonged to the more conservative group of doctors and sought only a few minor changes in the 1818 law. Although other committee members from the group of progressive doctors argued that a radical revision of medical legislation was necessary, and although they were supported by prominent professors (all from Amsterdam and Utrecht), the ministerial draft of legislation based on this report was rejected by Parliament. One committee member from the group of "modern" doctors then called for all medical professionals to join forces, asking, "How can we still remain active, now that the government does not want to do anything?" The answer was the establishment of the Dutch Association for the Promotion of Medicine (NMG).

The NMG was the first professional organization of doctors in the Netherlands after the guilds were abolished at the end of the eighteenth century. Its ideal was to establish medicine on a thoroughly scientific basis, and it demanded uniform standards in university education and in medical licensing. This demand for one and the same license for all doctors made the NMG officially an organization representing both graduates and nongraduates. In reality, though, the interests of these two groups were far from identical, a division reflected in the divergent viewpoints of the several local sections of the NMG. The founders of the organization, mostly reform-minded professors in Amsterdam and Utrecht with connections to higher governmental circles through their membership on state committees on the reorganization of medical law, functioned as a pressure group within the NMG and primarily served the interests of the graduate doctors. The scientific character of medicine was one of the arguments used by the NMG to stress the need for university-educated doctors. Although the progressive doctors' critique of the lamentable state of the organization of health care in the Netherlands may have been correct, their demands for change can also be interpreted as a strategy on the part of some graduates to assert their expertise in questions of health and disease. This point was made with particular eloquence by the aggressive Professor Mulder from Utrecht, a member of the NMG: "You, my gentlemen, are the experts here; your judgment, honestly and precisely expressed after thorough and extensive investigation, has to be elevated to law, and the States-General cannot but follow your judgment, because they are the nonexperts in medicine; they are there for the sake of unity, not to pass a judgment on things of which they have no knowledge."

This stress on education, the claim to expert knowledge, and demands for controls over education and licensing are among the elements of the process of professionalization that took place in Dutch medicine.[4] The strategic demand for a university education as the best form of medical training was clearly in the interest of the graduates. In this respect, this group profited from the persistent power of the radical young progressives in their ranks who were convinced that only scientific, rational knowledge could provide a valid foundation for all parts of medicine. The group's arguments referred not only to the use of rational methods, quantitative data, careful observation, and use of apparatus, but also implied a view of medicine as a unity of related subjects, not a collection of specialties. In this view, the basic science of medicine was physiology, which elucidated the general principles fundamental to the functioning of all life, just as Newtonian mechanics had become the basis of physics by elucidating the principles of the material world. The general laws of physiology, applicable to all life, united the medical sciences.

The changed conception of what medicine should be will be treated in the next section; here it is important to mention that this changing conception was reflected in the titles and content of contemporary journals, and in the take-over of their editorial boards by reform-minded doctors. Several new periodicals were also launched during the 1840s. In 1857 the NMG brought about a fusion of all the existing medical journals that shared its conception of scientific medicine, and the newly created *Dutch Journal of Medicine (Nederlands Tijdschrift voor Geneeskunde)* became the official organ of the NMG. In 1865, in the face of continuing demands from the board of the NMG, the authority of the medical professions was finally regulated. All medical students would be required henceforth to pass a state examination consisting of theoretical and clinical parts (the latter being new), which conveyed the right to the title of *Arts* (doctor) and authority to practice in all fields of medicine. At the same time, the requirement of writing a dissertation to acquire a license to practice was allowed to lapse.

All clinical schools were abolished, and though it was theoretically possible to take the examination without university training, in practice, the abolition of clinical schools signaled the final victory of the graduates. The requirements for the examination could be met only by attending the universities, or the *Athenaeum Illustre* in Amsterdam, which was not officially a university. Students of the *Athenaeum* could not pass the final examination in their own institute but had to take a state examination. The Amsterdam professors were so well represented on the state examination committee though that the *Athenaeum* had certainly, if reluctantly, to be taken seriously as a place for educating doctors by the three existing universities (Groningen, Utrecht, Leiden). In 1876, under unrelenting pressure of the powerful modernizers of medicine within the NMG, the *Athenaeum Illustre* became a university: the University of Amsterdam. As a result, medical education was completely localized in the universities, and the demands of the reformers were to a large extent met. Although this development had been strongly resisted by the long-established, conservative university of Leiden, the NMG board represented the more progressive group of doctors, of whom the Amsterdammers were an important part.

So, from 1876 onwards, the universities were obliged to offer clinical education to a large number of students, and professors were appointed in all clinical subjects. Slowly, the practices of the nongraduates were filled by graduates. The final regulation of medical authority and education meant not only a victory of the graduates over the nongraduates, but also the victory of a "modern" approach towards medicine over a conservative one. The idea of clinical medicine had become firmly established in the Netherlands by the last quarter of the nineteenth century.

CLINICAL MEDICINE

The origin of the modern concept of medicine, in which clinical medical practice plays such an important part, must be sought primarily in the flourishing medical centers of the first half of the century, and especially in Paris. Here, the combination of physical examination and autopsies was advocated as the only way to have valid knowledge of disease. Pathological anatomy and physical diagnostic methods, like auscultation, percussion, and measurement of body temperature, became central to medical training.[5] This approach, in which the clinic was vitally important, soon took root in other European cities with large hospitals. Vienna, in particular, became an outstanding medical center, and, besides the great French authorities like Bichat and Laennec, Skoda and Rokitansky acquired great authority in European medicine. Many Dutch doctors traveled to both Paris and Vienna after having finished their studies.

The influence of these schools can be traced, for example, in the career of Jan van Geuns, who was appointed by the Amsterdam City Council in 1847 as a professor of forensic medicine and general pathology in the *Athenaeum Illustre*. Previously, professors there were expected to provide only a theoretical education in medicine. Students had almost no opportunity to apply their knowledge in actual practice during their studies. The clinical school in Amsterdam, which did possess a reasonable hospital, educated the nonacademic doctors and was forbidden ground for the *Atheneum* professors. Van Geuns, however, agreed to accept his professorship only on condition that "I be given the opportunity to relate the study of pathology to observations at the sickbed, and this not only for reasons of personal practice, but especially for the sake of education and science." In fact, he found support in the reports of foreign visitors who had questioned the absence of links between medical education and hospitals in the Netherlands. After an initial refusal, the city authorities and the board of governors of the clinical school hospital finally accepted his condition. In his inaugural lecture, he further elaborated the relation between medical theory and practice:

> As soon as the fruits of scientific investigation are taken up by practical medicine, as soon as the development and course of the investigations of science exercise their influences on the art, so that the eye is directed in its observations and the acts of the doctor are governed by theory, the separation between theory and practice in the further development of science becomes dangerous.
>
> The fusion [of theory and practice] has to be reestablished with new force by science, which must provide us with the objectives of our searching; it must allow us to recognize distinctly the direction that will lead us to those objec-

tives. The word in which this all comes together is: medicine must be an independent natural science.[6]

Van Geuns put all his energy into attempts to create the scientific medicine he sketched in his inaugural lecture. It was he who introduced auscultation and percussion, the so-called physical methods of clinical investigation, and the thermometer into the clinic.

In the second half of the century, however, developments in Germany became the focus of attention of the medical world. Young German doctors were reacting strongly against the speculative theories in the romantic tradition most prevalent in Germany at the beginning of the nineteenth century. They built on the accomplishments of the Paris and Vienna schools, but objected to their purely anatomical approach. They put much more emphasis on the study of the process of the disease than on its locally visible end products. Disease, according to this view, should be seen as a disturbance of basic body functions, and for these to be known, medicine had to identify the general laws and principles that regulated the process in the body. Physiology, consequently, was vitally important. In France, Claude Bernard had to fight the powerful clinicians who were not prepared to give up their strongly hospital-based medicine for a laboratory-based physiology. Germany, where the new role of full-time professional scientist developed, provided a more fertile ground for this new conception of medicine.[7]

The new views on clinical medicine, in which physiological pathology had become the most important field of study, began to be felt throughout Europe and the United States. In the Netherlands, this can be traced, for example, in Van Geuns' attempts to establish a laboratory. Largely as a result of his efforts, in 1855 a physiological pathological laboratory was set up in an old kitchen of the clinical school. In 1858 he was able to persuade the city council to provide the money for an extra professorship in physiology in order to assure education in that part of the subject "that rests more immediately on chemical and physical experiments."[8]

In Utrecht, Donders, who already enjoyed an international reputation as a physiologist, was granted a professorship in this subject in 1852. He was also one of the representatives of the "new medicine" and was active in the NMG. He, too, was convinced of the need for a strong link between practice and theory, and he combined his experimental research involving the physiology of sight in animals with his practice as an ophthalmologist in an Utrecht eye-clinic for the poor, especially created for him with private money. Except for Donders' laboratory and clinic, the medical faculty of Utrecht University was poorly equipped and had a very small hospital. The same was true for Groningen, where the university was, in fact, constantly in danger of being closed down because of the lack of students. In Leiden, where discussions with the city authorities about the building of a proper hospital went on for decades, it was an uphill struggle as well.

The new German conception of clinical medicine rejected ontological concepts of disease: illness was understood as a disturbance or deregulation of
the basic processes in the body. Virchow, the promoter of clinical science in
Germany, defined illness as follows: "All diseases can ultimately be traced
back to active or passive disturbances of bigger or smaller assemblies of vital
elements, the performance of which changes according to the state of their
molecular composition and therefore depends on the physical and chemical
changes of their contents." Virchow's definition elucidates the importance of
physical and chemical processes in the body. Physiology, looked upon as a
model discipline resembling the natural sciences, was to unravel the basic
process of life and, by experiment, identify the laws according to which they
worked. Virchow possessed great authority among progressive Dutch doctors.
As Leopold Lehmann, a reader in obstetrics in the Amsterdam clinical school
and one of the founders of the NMG, stated in 1863, "The brilliant Virchow,
who as a result of his investigations and experiments has expressed and introduced as the now predominant principle in science this great thought about
the healthy and diseased state of life, i.e., that phenomena of disease are
phenomena of life, in principle just as lawlike and necessary as the expres-
sions of the whole body."[9] He stressed the status of clinical science in relation
to physiology by emphasizing the relation between medical knowledge and
clinical practice:

> Physiology may be the basis for medicine, but it does not always follow the
> right road, and results gathered outside the body have often been applied too
> lightheartedly to phenomena in the living organism. Great physiologists, more-
> over, are seldom good doctors at the sick bed, and no wonder, since where the
> clinic has disappeared and only the laboratory governs, no medicine can flour-
> ish rightly. Not everything may be offered to the cult of facts under the flag of
> the auxiliary sciences: it [rational therapy] has to be found, based on clinical ex-
> perience, supported by experiment and induction; it has to be applied and to be
> controlled by statistics.[10]

The emphasis on physiology as a basic science and on clinical practice was
of vital importance, for medical science went hand in hand with the strong
conviction that human beings were actually capable of influencing physiological processes by controlling the physical and chemical factors:

> The organic processes of the human organism are no less subject to our power
> than those of organic nature. Just as one can force the soil to produce one har-
> vest or another when one knows the conditions of its fertility and the means
> that influence it, so it will also be possible to control the functions of some or-
> gans, to limit the pathological processes in their course and to stop them.[11]

The conditions under which the idea of clinical science arose in the Netherlands show some similarities to those in Germany, but they also show some
important differences. In the first place, both in Germany and in the Nether-

lands, the progressive doctors were young, which made for a generational conflict with the older, more traditional group. However, the traditional views the modernizers reacted against were different in the two countries. Although romanticism was a strongly established tradition in Germany, in the Netherlands it was much less extreme, leading some historians to speak of eclecticism rather than romanticism. Moreover, although the social and political instability of the 1840s and 1850s was great in both countries, the Dutch progressives did not engage in political action to the same extent as the Germans.[12] The conscious link in Germany between reform in science and medicine and reform in society was not present in the Netherlands in the same form. The objective of the Dutch reformers was to assert their authority on questions of health, education, and the licensing of doctors, and to take this authority over from the state. This was the content of their political struggle and the basis for the establishment of the NMG. Initially, the government regarded the establishment and the articles of the association as an attempt to resist the legal authority of the state, but such "misunderstandings" were soon clarified:

> The breeding of revolutionary principles is something never thought of in our Association. Moreover, nothing has been further removed from our Association ... than the pursuit of political influence. On the contrary, one of its greatest advantages is that it stands outside all politics, that no political orientations exist for it. It only strives for improvements it is qualified to judge and that are of equal importance for all parties, for all directions.[13]

Indeed, although some of the reformers united in the NMG did engage in more political and social debates, the fact that the group that promoted the ideal of scientific medicine had organized the NMG primarily as a professional organization gave the ideal of reform in medicine, as it was picked up from Germany, a particular coloring, one linked to professional interests.

THE IDEAL OF CLINICAL SCIENCES IN OBSTETRICS

Having sketched the institutional and ideological changes in general terms, we can now turn to obstetrics, where we find the same ideas about clinical science. Such ideas were expressed in the lectures of Leopold Lehmann, the Amsterdam obstetrician, for example, in his inaugural lecture of 1865, in which he mentioned the status of obstetrics as a separate scientific discipline within medicine, and stated that the distance between the art and the science of obstetrics had been bridged when "better knowledge about the physiology and the mechanism of birth filled the gap and gave the discipline a truly scientific character." He traced the origin of this idea to Germany, "from which the clear light that now continues to elucidate obstetrics as an exact science par excellence has spread over all the countries of Europe."

Similar statements were made by other professors of obstetrics in their inaugural lectures. They all stressed the unity of medicine, but at the same time sought to legitimate its independent status as a scientific discipline by recalling its long-standing tradition and its famous representatives in science, with special reference to Germany. The names of Schroeder, Ruge, Michaelis, Naegele, and Boer were often mentioned. Indeed, obstetrics was a specialty with a history, and not only an art or skill. It was a subject taught in the universities as early as the eighteenth century, but the teaching had been purely theoretical and not given special attention. Surgery, in combination with which it was taught, was thought to have higher status.

In practice, normal deliveries had been almost exclusively the concern of midwives, who were obliged to summon the help of a man-midwife or a surgeon in complicated cases, since midwives were not allowed to use instruments or perform operations. The graduate *doctores artis obstetricae* were called in for help only in exceptional cases. As the practice of midwifery came to be more strictly regulated by law and the *doctores* had to take care of the education and supervision of midwives, the need for more practical training soon became apparent. As a result, in 1848, Abraham Simon Thomas was appointed in Leiden to the first chair of obstetrics and gynecology separate from surgery. Elsewhere, the chair remained a combination of surgery and obstetrics. The clinical schools taught surgery and obstetrics at a practical level, but here also the two fields were combined. Amsterdam was an exception, with Lehmann appointed in 1848 as reader in obstetrics.

With the introduction of the 1865 law, clinical professors of the clinical subjects were appointed at all the universities. The clinical schools, as we have seen, did not meet the new criteria for medical education and were closed, except for the Amsterdam school, which maintained a high standard and a good reputation. Eventually it merged with the *Athenaeum Illustre*, with which it already had strong links because many of the professors had appointments in both places. As a result of this merger, the *Athenaeum* had an extraordinarily advantageous position. In order to enlarge the practical training of students by assisting in home births under the supervision of midwives (the so-called *secours à domicile*), the university professors of Leiden, Utrecht, and Groningen had to make special arrangements with the midwives. The university clinics were too small. In their inaugural lectures, professors of obstetrics from 1865 onwards pleaded for extension of the obstetrical clinics. When in 1895, Treub, the successor of Simon Thomas in Leiden, was offered the chair in Amsterdam, he accepted immediately, because Amsterdam had a larger obstetrical clinic, gynecological clinic, and polyclinic.

The new professors of obstetrics appointed in 1865, all representatives of "modern" medicine, took their educational tasks very seriously, convinced as they were that only this new approach to medicine could provide the rational knowledge necessary for a doctor to treat his patients adequately. The emphasis on teaching is also apparent in the effort the new professors put into the writing of textbooks. Simon Thomas wrote a small textbook; his successor, Treub, published a two-volume text on gynecology; Van der Mey, the successor of Lehmann in Amsterdam, began a major textbook on obstetrics that was completed by Treub, who completely reworked the third edition into a new textbook. Sänger in Groningen also published a handbook on obstetrics.

This emphasis on education raises the questions of how these propagators of modern medicine approached their newly established positions in the university, how they perceived their roles as clinical scientists, and what this meant in terms of the relative emphasis on teaching and research. The Dutch obstetricians did produce certain clinical research results that were also known outside of the Netherlands. Simon Thomas, professor in Leiden from 1848 to 1886, gained recognition for his study of the unevenly narrowed pelvis, inspired by the great work of Michaelis on the mensuration of the pelvis. Simon Thomas introduced this work in the Netherlands, but could not approach the enormous number of measurements that Michaelis had made in order to make his classifications and establish his concept of the normal pelvis. Another contribution of Simon Thomas was in the field of gynecology, in which he published an account of twelve cases of ovariotomy, then a rather novel operation, and a new technique for the closing of the uterus after Caesarean section. Halbertsma, professor in Groningen in 1866–67 and from 1867 onwards in Utrecht, became known outside the country for his work on eclampsia. Sänger, professor in Groningen from 1867 to 1898, acquired a reputation for his work on vaginal uterus extirpation.

All this work, however, dealt largely with special cases, and only a few descriptions were required before a scientific report could be published. The Dutch could not keep pace with the experimental research that became so predominant from about 1850, especially in Germany. In the 1860s, German research dealt chiefly with physiological measurements; in the 1870s with the role of the kidneys in pregnancy and with the innervation of the uterus; in the 1880s on pelvic measurements with instruments, ectopic pregnancies, and the physiology of the placenta and the fetus. Only Halbertsma in Utrecht made contributions in this area, no doubt profiting from the experimental climate there and from Donders' well-equipped physiological laboratory.

Yet it remained virtually impossible to match the major clinical studies from abroad, in which new theories and experimentally established hypotheses could be put to the test. This lack of research activity is also reflected in the articles that appeared in the *Dutch Journal for Obstetrics and Gynecology (NTvVG)*. This journal, established in 1889 by the Dutch Association for Gynecology, long suffered a precarious existence. Its first two volumes mainly contained articles from the Leiden and Amsterdam clinics, but the number of such articles gradually declined from twenty-four in its first two years to nine in the last two years of the century. From the third year onwards, it was filled primarily with the contributions of doctors with private practices. A strong orientation towards German research is also visible in the content of the articles before 1900. Of all the references, 55–80 percent were to German sources, 5–35 percent to French sources, and 4–20 percent to Dutch sources. Gynecological articles, and especially those on operations, formed the main part of the journal in the first years, but from 1893, they gradually gave way to articles on the physiology of pregnancy or the female organs, or on complicated deliveries and pelvimetry.

The enthusiasm for gynecological operations was so great that some doctors spoke of the "operating fury" that had taken over. By the end of the century, the growing concern about this development was reflected in the inaugural lectures of professors. Treub, for example, in a lecture on "The danger of contemporary gynecology," warned against careless diagnosis and casual decisions to operate. The connection between gynecology and obstetrics was emphasized, as was the relevance of nonoperative gynecology.

Another available source that allows us to reconstruct the nature and amount of scientific work produced in the Netherlands consists of dissertations. The publication of regular discussion in the *NTvVG* of all dissertations published from 1889–95 is of help here. With an average of some five dissertations per year, there were not many to review. During this six-year period, there were no dissertations from Groningen, only one from Utrecht, seven from Amsterdam, and twenty-six from Leiden, written under the supervision of Treub. Almost all dealt with theoretical considerations based on literature, with descriptions of a very limited number of cases, or with a report of the clinic over a certain period. The case descriptions, often of one or two observations made while working as an assistant in the university clinic, were augmented with some observations from private practice, which was usually established after the assistantship, or with some reports of cases treated by the professor or other doctors.

Thus we have to conclude that during the nineteenth century, no research tradition in obstetrics was established in the Netherlands as had been the case in Germany, where the prevailing ideas seem to have been similar. This was so despite the fact that Dutch doctors were convinced by the idea of clinical science and had promoted this idea against more conservative currents by emphasizing scientific knowledge as the basis for the furtherance of medicine; that they had won their fight for a medical education completely located in the university and intrinsically connected with scientific research; and that many prominent natural scientists were working in the Dutch universities and favored a climate conducive to scientific research. Why was this so? To answer it, we must examine clinical practice, which is of such vital importance for clinical research. Since Germany served as a model for the Netherlands, a comparison of the conditions of clinical practice in the two countries should be helpful in elucidating those factors in clinical practice that are important in explaining the differences.

THE CONDITIONS OF CLINICAL PRACTICE IN THE NETHERLANDS AND GERMANY COMPARED

In Germany, there were more, larger, and better-equipped clinics than in the Netherlands. These provided more opportunities for research and education. In the Netherlands, there were no trained nurses: nursing personnel were recruited from penal institutions, and the descriptions of the deplorable and unhygienic circumstances of patients lying in dark, unventilated rooms, having to bribe nurses to obtain the food and wine to which they were entitled, speak for themselves. These circumstances were not very favorable to clinical investigations. It was not until 1883 that training for nurses was introduced in the Amsterdam clinic, the biggest in the country, not surprisingly by German "sisters." No qualified people could be found in the Netherlands to set up nursing care in the hospital. Since the 1870s, when private hospitals with proper furnishings and nursing had been established, the deplorable Amsterdam university clinic had found itself competing with these for patients. Moreover, in 1871, everyone entering the hospital, patients and visitors alike, had to pay for admission, and when a patient died, relatives had to pay for the removal of the corpse. The medical professors tried to overcome this rule by distributing their visiting cards for free admittance. Although this situation improved during the last quarter of the century, an 1882 hospital board report about the state of the hospitals described the situation as completely intolerable.

Another difference between the two countries was their clinical laboratories. Führbringer, a professor of anatomy in Amsterdam of German origin, complained about the state of the laboratories, as did his successor and fellow countryman, Ruge. Sometimes professors threatened to accept jobs elsewhere, or raised private funds to set up special clinics. A colleague of Donders in Amsterdam refused to accept a professorship in ophthalmology in 1894 without a better-equipped clinic, something accomplished by a huge legacy.

As the examples of Führbringer and Ruge make clear, the orientation of Dutch medicine towards Germany was at that time apparent not only in references to German literature and to German medical scientists, but also in the fact that a number of doctors went to Germany to study and work in the universities there, and that Germans were appointed as professors in the Netherlands.[14] Despite legislation to the effect that no foreigners should be appointed as professors, several, in fact, were.[15] For example, Hertz became professor of special pathological anatomy in 1867. He was not only German, but had been proposed for the professorship by Virchow himself. Hertz actively promoted clinical education in Amsterdam. Kuhn, Van Geuns' successor appointed in 1877, was a Dutchman, but he had worked in Germany with Virchow and Von Recklinghausen. None of the Germans stayed very long, however, and most of them eventually returned to their own country.

It is likely that the situation of the clinics played a role here. This can be illustrated in the case of obstetrics. As J. Veit, a German professor in Leiden from 1896 to 1903, described the situation, "The clinical material was small, even smaller than in my private practice in Berlin." Veit started his own research, "making use of the only material that was available to me in sufficient quantities, i.e., placentas." During his time in Leiden, he saw the number of deliveries rise from 128 to 165 per year, while cases in the gynecological clinic rose from 189 to 300, and in the gynecological polyclinic from 248 to 590. After his professorship in Leiden, he accepted a chair in Erlangen, and, a year later, one in Halle, "where I can make use of ample material, i.e., in the obstetrical clinic approximately 700 cases, the gynecological clinic more than 1,000 cases, and in the gynecological polyclinic 3,500 cases." Veit was not the only one who left. Döderlein, appointed in Groningen in 1897, left for Germany again after only three months; Güsserow in Utrecht stayed only a year (1867–68); and the proposed German successor of Lehmann in Amsterdam, Zweifel, did not even accept the chair. That all these were Germans is remarkable.

In the previous section, we saw the extent to which the Dutch modern medical scientists were oriented towards Germany. This orientation is so overwhelming that complaints about the Germanization of the language and of Dutch medicine began to be voiced in the *Nederlands Tijdschrift voor Geneeskunde* (NTG). This last point was raised by Treub in his protest against Döderlein's appointment, which caused a break in contact with Veit, and accounts for the fact that the Germans stayed away from the third international congress of gynecology and obstetrics held in Amsterdam in 1899.

Veit's report of his professorship in Leiden also contains a striking complaint about the closing of the clinic during student vacations. Veit initiated a discussion in the NTG to have this state of affairs changed. He was struck by the extent to which his Dutch colleagues viewed the clinics more as training grounds for students than as places in which to do research; and, of course, education was the major concern of the clinical disciplines. After 1865, they were suddenly confronted with a large number of students who needed practical training.

As we have seen, one of the major difficulties of the obstetricians was their lack of clinical material. Amsterdam was an exception to this, and more research should have been done there, where Lehmann, the promoter of scientific obstetrics, was a professor. As we have already seen, however, the Amsterdam clinic was in a deplorable state with respect to hygiene and nursing. This condition also extended to the Amsterdam maternity clinic, which after 1867 was housed in a new larger building with 106 beds. There were several discussions between the faculty and the city authorities about its closure, as well as contemporary brochures. It appears that of the 106 beds, an average of twenty to twenty-four were occupied by pregnant women, while the rest were filled with sick children, sufferers from eye diseases, and pa-

tients recovering from surgery. According to another report, 615 fewer
women came to the new clinic during the first six years of its existence than
had come to the old clinic in the course of the previous six years. Moreover,
Lehmann was strongly opposed to the idea of puerperal fever as a contagious
disease: in fact, he followed Virchow, for whom the idea of contagion resem-
bled an ontological conception of disease. This meant that the university clinic
was frequently ravaged by the disease. The mortality among women in the
clinic increased from 4 percent in the years 1865–76, to 8 percent in 1877,
to 14 percent in the first few months of 1878. This was one reason why the
city authorities closed the clinic in May of that year. Women feared to go
there to deliver their babies, and only the extremely poor, who could not even
afford to pay a midwife, would go.

Although Semmelweis had convincingly demonstrated the effect of antiseptic measures on the death rate in maternity clinics in 1846, many "modern"
doctors refused to believe in the contagious origins of illness.[16] As Catharina
Van Tusschenbroek remarked in her study on aseptic obstetrics in the Netherlands, "It was Virchow's authority in the Netherlands that stood in the way
of Semmelweis's acknowledgment." Until his death, Lehmann remained a convinced disbeliever. His physiological studies may indeed have been a major
factor contributing to the propagation of this deadly disease, since, for example, he apparently used the same thermometer for healthy and sick women to
measure the temperature in the uterus before, during, and after delivery.

After Lehmann's death in 1880, his successor, Van der Mey, brought down
the death rate in the clinic in a few years through the introduction of anti-
and aseptic measures. Furthermore, although he contributed some articles to
the first issues of *NTvVG*, his energy seems to have been directed more
to improvement of the conditions for the development of gynecology in
Amsterdam, a subject that had been somewhat neglected by Lehmann. Moreover, moving the university clinic to another hospital meant that for a while,
part of the department was housed in an old canal house, a situation far from
favorable to clinical research.

Compared with Germany, clinical practice in obstetrics in the Netherlands
was characterized by small hospitals, bad nursing conditions, little clinical material, and badly equipped clinical laboratories. Even in the relatively favorable
situation of Amsterdam, conditions were such that clinical research could not
begin to develop. More importantly, the Dutch clinics remained primarily oriented to the education of students, a situation brought about by a conception
of scientific medicine that was shaped by the professionalization process.

THE INSTITUTIONAL SETTING OF OBSTETRICS

The availability of clinical material was an important way in which Dutch
obstetrical practice differed from that in Germany, but it can only be one element in an explanation of the failure to develop a Dutch obstetrical research

tradition comparable to that in Germany. The discussion of the process of professionalization among the Dutch doctors showed that there was a strong emphasis on medical education. Demands for university training were not only to raise the level of knowledge of doctors, but also to assert the special status of medical knowledge. Before 1876, this argument played an important role in the professionalization strategy of the graduate doctors in their competition against the nongraduates. As a result, education was strongly emphasized within the university setting of clinical medicine. Clinical science thus came to be equated more with scientific education in the clinic than with research. Apparently, the idea of clinical science as a "real" science was still such a charged issue that Treub, talking in 1899 about clinical obstetrical science in a lecture to the NMG, remarked: "I don't have to excuse myself for talking of clinical science, do I?"

As already noted, this preoccupation with education is not only present in almost every inaugural lecture and voiced repeatedly in public speeches and reports, but also apparent in the fact that so many obstetricians put their efforts into the writing of textbooks. Still, the doctors were not totally unaware of the problems of combining research with education, as is apparent from a statement made at the yearly lecture to the assembly of the NMG in 1888:

> In the question of the education of doctors the great difficulty is that we are all convinced that science, above all, should provide a basis for education, but that we do not know exactly how to make room for pure science in education without failing to meet the demands of practice. This difficulty has been present in our Association for years. Here also the question has been: what place should we give to science, the pursuit of which has been the explicit objective of the Association?[17]

The doctors were not alone in looking upon the university in this manner, and we need to consider the broader set of expectations for the Dutch universities in the latter part of the nineteenth century.

At least as far as medicine was concerned, the universities were seen primarily as training grounds for students and not as places in which to do research. The loss of students, for example, meant that the very existence of the university was endangered, as in the case of Groningen. In Amsterdam as late as the 1890s, the city council proposed closing down the university because it cost too much money for too few students, and only served as "an institute for hobbyists" or as "an unnecessary, reckless, irresponsible luxury."[18] This was said at a time when Van't Hoff and Van der Waals in the same university had established international scientific reputations as researchers. The extent to which similar problems were faced in other sciences is not clear. This question remains to be answered by studies of the history of the development of Dutch universities. That the state was reluctant to provide the necessary money to extend and improve laboratories is apparent from the

many pleas for funds for this purpose, which were rejected by the authorities
with skeptical remarks about pure science.

In his report to the NMG on the comparison between higher medical education in Germany and the Netherlands, Treub stated that "the clinical laboratories are generally much better in Germany than in the Netherlands," and he
also called attention to another important difference, the number of assistants. Not only was the scientific medical staff much larger in Germany, but
they also held better positions and were better paid. In the Netherlands before 1879, the assistants to the professors were students of medicine, and although from that year they were required to be doctors who had completed
their studies, salaries were so low that it was hard to keep anybody for more
than one or two years. In fact, even the professors were poorly paid. When
Donders, for example, left his teaching job in a school in The Hague for a university chair in Utrecht, his salary was cut by more than half, so that he had
to do translations in the evenings to support his family.

Another factor was the disincentive to produce dissertations. With the introduction of the title of *Arts* (doctor), the need to write a dissertation in
order to graduate and acquire a license to practice had disappeared. Furthermore, since there was little incentive after 1865 in the form of senior posts,
extra pay, or professional status, the number of dissertations remained small.
The fact that it was relatively easy to acquire the title of "doctor" in some
German states or Belgium (where the writing of a dissertation was not required) also dampened enthusiasm for graduating with a dissertation in the
Netherlands.

> The fact that the public makes no distinction between those who have and
> those who have not written a doctoral dissertation and, moreover, that all who
> return after a short trip abroad with a German "Doctor's diploma" can carry
> this title with impunity, may serve as an excuse. But we have to fear that in
> this way a title which for centuries conveyed a high status in social life will be-
> come stigmatized as a foolish eccentricity, probably even a ridiculous arrogance
> to make colleagues envious. *Caveant consules.*[19]

Looking somewhat more closely at the dissertations that were written in
obstetrics, we see that these still had the traditional character of theoretical
pieces of work, mostly based on studies of the literature without clinical research. It is characteristic that most of them were written in Leiden, and almost none in Amsterdam, which should have been the most favorable place
for clinical research. The medical dissertation in the Netherlands was still located in the historical context of these two universities: conservative Leiden,
where a graduate degree in medicine was traditionally based on a theoretical
work, and modern Amsterdam, where there was no tradition of writing a dissertation at all, since the university-to-be lacked the *ius examinandi* until
1877. Here, too, one of the obvious ways to do research, namely in the

framework of graduate study, was inhibited by the fact that no new institutional incentives to write dissertations were created. The thesis preserved its historical form, even though its function had lost its traditional meaning under the new legislation, and was accorded no new significance by the creation of careers in science. In fact, there existed hardly any opportunities for a scientific career: "one cannot blame . . . the young doctor if his eagerness to do scientific work is not very great, when there is no future, in whatever form, connected with it."[20]

The lack of opportunity to do scientific work was also given as a reason why foreigners often occupied chairs in the universities. It seemed that no sufficiently qualified Dutch candidates were available: "Our medical Faculties do produce many skillful people . . . but they offer the students little or no opportunity to engage in long, continuing scientific research, and this is one of the reasons why almost every time a Chair has to be filled anew, the choice among our young doctors . . . is only a very limited one."[21]

Both the loss of the social function of the dissertation and the fact that no new careers in science emerged in the Dutch universities contributed to the low number of dissertations produced. This, together with the differences between Leiden and Amsterdam, indicates that the university maintained its traditional position with respect to medicine; although the idea of clinical research was introduced, the university did not function as a research institute.

One last issue to be considered in the discussion of institutional arrangements is the size of the country. In the first place, this factor is, of course, responsible up to a point for the size of hospitals and the number of patients. If we again make the comparison with Germany, we see that in the last quarter of the nineteenth century, there were twenty universities in Germany with twenty-one women's clinics (Berlin had two clinics), all built after 1860, providing the doctors there with 10,000 deliveries and an equal number of gynecological cases every year. In addition to professors and assistants, there were doctors working voluntarily in fourteen of the clinics in 1893. Moreover, every university also had obstetrical and gynecological polyclinics. By comparison, the Netherlands had four university women's clinics, three of them with polyclinics, with a total of some 600 deliveries a year until the beginning of the 1880s. From 1880 until the end of the century, the number rose to approximately 850 a year. Amsterdam represented by far the highest number of deliveries, from 350 to some 500 a year by the end of the century.

What is to be noted here is not so much the size of each clinic; rather the point is that the overall clinical activity, the number of professorships, and the number of doctors involved in university clinics all created in Germany an atmosphere that must have been quite different from the homely, friendly atmosphere in the Netherlands. Again, we can find indications in support of this hypothesis in institutional arrangements. The Amsterdam Gynaecological Association was established in 1887 by the Amsterdam professor of obstetrics and gynecology, Van der Mey, and some doctors with private practices, all graduates in obstetrics and gynecology. Their objective was to talk about "special issues in their field of science," and the association was rebaptized the Dutch Association of Gynaecology (*Nederlandsche Gynaecologische Vereniging*, NGV).

Treub in Leiden and Van der Mey in Amsterdam were especially active in the association. At meetings, usually with no more than seven or eight members present, they would examine patients under narcosis, show preparations, or lecture about difficult deliveries and operations. Foreign articles and books were also discussed. "In accordance with the jovial character that typified our meetings, we often examined patients difficult to diagnose, and all who were present took part in the discussion." Furthermore: "Eating together, a thing that sociable doctors fortunately have always appreciated, seduced us in 1901 not to meet at all in July, but instead to have a feast for no other reason, as is mentioned in the minutes, than that summer is here."[22]

Apparently, the attempts that were made towards the end of the century to change the character of the association were not really successful even in 1901, but we do gradually see an awareness of its "kind-hearted conviviality" and a desire to change it. The organization of the Third International Congress of Gynecology and Obstetrics in Amsterdam by the NGV contributed to this, as did the decision to publish the reports of the meetings of the association in the *Zentralblatt für Gynecologie*. "All this indicates that our Association is going through a metamorphosis; the small, convivial Amsterdam circle of years gone by will develop into a real, official Association. . . . We should not want to go back to those bygone days. . . . It [the Association] can become a scientific and ethical force to the benefit of the whole country."[23]

The journal of the association also suffered from the fact that so few people were involved: "Once again it has to be stated openly here that more than once the editorial board had to deal with such a dearth of copy that it was not always possible to publish a volume in time."[24] Indeed, foreign obstetricians wondered about the fact that the association could keep a specialist journal going in such a small linguistic area. We have to wonder whether the small, convivial, circle-of-friends atmosphere that typified Dutch obstetrics could have influenced the attitude of the obstetricians towards research. Reading the minutes, the reports, and the retrospects, we get a picture of hard-working, skillful, individually operating doctors who liked to lecture, report, and discuss their practical work in these informal meetings. Daily problems in obstetrical practice took up much of their attention. Remembering his time in Leiden, Veit said:

> I profited especially from encounters with very brilliant physicists in this work [on placentas], by whose information I hoped to find a way to understand fetal metabolism better. In this way I studied the osmotic pressure with Dekhuyzen and the intrusion of flocks in the bloodstream with Hoffman, and so I got into

the field in which I still work, and never would I have been able to develop it if my encounters with Kamerling Onnes and others in Leiden had not been so easy.[25]

If we consider why Dutch obstetricians did not seek the same cooperation with natural scientists as Veit did, we can only guess that the particular "provincial" setting of Dutch obstetrical science was an important factor. Even as late as 1920, the members of the association could only sigh over the loss of the regular contributions of a pathological anatomist, who left their circle when he was appointed professor. If we compare this attitude with Veit's active search for cooperation, we can only marvel at such inertia.

To conclude: the institutional setting of Dutch obstetrics in the nineteenth century was unfavorable to the growth of research activities in this field. This situation resulted from the particular circumstances under which the process of professionalization took place, which strongly emphasized the educational side of scientific medicine, as well as from the fact that the traditional climate in the universities remained much the same after the reorganization of medical education in 1865, which contributed to the "provincial" atmosphere that prevailed in Dutch obstetrics.

CONCLUSION

The struggle for professionalization within Dutch medicine and the strategy adopted by the reformers gave a particular emphasis to the idea of scientific medicine: an emphasis on education, on the provision of knowledge for use in practice. This background of professionalization, which characterized Dutch medicine up to the late 1870s, served to unite the graduate doctors in their competition with other practitioners. This is diametrically opposed to the situation in Germany, where scientific medicine was heavily influenced by the ideas of Von Humboldt, who emphasized pure research as the main objective of the scientist, and the freedom of teaching and the unity of teaching and research as the leading principles of the universities.[26] The influence of these ideas created an atmosphere at the German universities that was very much oriented to research, and it became the condition for the establishment of the "research imperative"[27] connected with another professionalization process, that of university teachers. There was competition among medical scientists not for acquiring professional independence as a doctor, but for acquiring status as a researcher.[28] The concept of scientific medicine thus had a double significance for its Dutch promoters, embodying both the ideal of what medicine should be (taken over from Germany) and a sense of the professionalization strategies developed within their own Dutch context.

The outcome of their struggle was the establishment of medical training in the universities, which provided them (bearing in mind their concept of medical science) with conditions that appeared favorable to those who looked to the establishment of a research tradition. Indeed it must have seemed so to the German bearers of a comparable tradition who came to the Dutch universities, but achievements in research were limited, and the Germans usually returned home disappointed. A university setting and an unquestioned belief that medicine "ought to be a science" were not sufficient conditions for the establishment of a research tradition. Comparison of the situation in Germany with that in the Netherlands suggests several possible reasons for the differences.

First, although the ideal of clinical science in the Netherlands, as in Germany, was promoted by a group of young enthusiastic doctors reacting against a conservative and romantic approach to medicine in a context of great social instability, the romantic tradition was far less deeply rooted in the Netherlands. The milder reaction among the Dutch doctors is thus understandable. They were also less involved in social and political reform than their German counterparts, and Dutch attempts to change medicine were not part of a broader movement of social reform, as was the case in Germany. This broader political involvement seems to have been a source of strength to the German group (as well as an influence on their intellectual development). The Dutch doctors, in contrast, were more closely bound to a narrow conception of professional interests, involving essentially the search for control over education and licensing.

Second, for the German visitors there were, of course, no such ideological constraints. For them, more simply, failure and disappointment can be seen more in material terms. An important element here was the lack of clinical material. Beyond this, the research-minded doctors, notably the German professors, came into conflict with a university system that seems in general not to have been adapted to the new research orientation emerging in Europe and the United States. There was no perceived linkage between the requirements of medical education, on the one hand, and the pursuit of medical knowledge on the other. The Dutch doctors who had spoken so strongly for training were, in fact, likely to be judged both in terms of their capacities as healers and by their educational efforts (including the writing of textbooks).

It is important to stress that Dutch universities did not develop a "research imperative" as in Germany, an ethos that strongly emphasized the production of original research. There was no need to write a research-based dissertation in order to obtain an academic post, nor was there the possibility of making a reputation based on research achievements. These stimuli were lacking. The possibility of a research career has been put forward as an important precondition for the beginning of research, and the absence of any institutional encouragement must have been a major inhibition in the Netherlands.[29]

Third, and strongly related to this, was the passive, laissez-faire attitude of the state and the lack of any governmental stimulation. This was in marked contrast to Germany. Laboratories in the Netherlands were small and badly equipped, and resources were not easy to acquire. There was no recognition of the need to provide resources or the need to stimulate new fields of science.

Fourth, according to some authors, competition was an important factor in the development of German medical science. This competition was essentially lacking in the Netherlands, despite the discussions between the Leiden (Treub) and Amsterdam (Van der Mey) professors about the "international" character of their respective clinics. Treub refers here to his contacts with gynecologists in Paris, whereas Van der Mey refers to the variety of nationalities among his patients. Although Treub was proud of his role in the Third International Congress on Gynecology and Obstetrics, this was, in fact, due less to his research output than to his personality, his ability to speak foreign languages, and the wide scope of his foreign contacts. It was the result of the state of mind that still existed, which promoted group feeling rather than competitiveness. This, together with the fact that research reputations were simply not to be made in the Netherlands, is clearly a major explanatory factor.

Finally, the particular atmosphere of the Dutch obstetrical community contributed to the lack of research. This seems to be a necessary independent factor: there is no obvious reason why small groups of scientists in friendly contact with one another should not produce high-quality research. The contrast with the physical sciences is, after all, striking, for they too suffered from the same lack of resources and career opportunities, and from state indifference. Even the lack of clinical material is insufficient to give a satisfying explanation. What seems crucial here is that despite an allegiance to "clinical science," the Dutch university doctors did not see themselves as scientists, but rather as broadly oriented, all-knowing, classically schooled, and high-status members of society. Any explanation of the slow development of Dutch obstetric research in the nineteenth century must clearly be composed of a variety of interrelated elements: professional and political ideologies (the latter restricting the role of the state), themselves understandable in sociocultural terms, and the manifestations of all this in the relevant institutions of Dutch society.

THE PRESENT DAY: DISCUSSION AND EPILOG

This picture of Dutch research in obstetrics at the end of the nineteenth century that has emerged in the foregoing account is a rather bleak one. In the intervening years, things have changed. Hospitals are bigger, and there is no longer a lack of "clinical material"; nursing care is of good quality, and laboratories are well equipped. There is generous state support for research. On the other hand, certain other aspects of Dutch obstetrics have remained surprisingly similar for a long time, including its small size and uniform character. Until the late 1950s, there were only four university departments of obstetrics and gynecology and only four chairs for these combined subjects.[30]

Education also long remained a major concern for obstetricians. In the 1930s, the regulation of medical specialties demanded a great deal of attention to training and education, as did the revisions of the requirements for obstetrical training in the 1940s and 1960s. An additional concern remained the education and training of future general practitioners, given their considerable share in the management of deliveries. They, too, had to be taught the principles and practice of obstetrics.[31] Finally, obstetricians were also involved in the training of midwives and maternity home-care assistants, who were all part of the Dutch system of health care surrounding pregnancy and delivery.

Another aspect of Dutch obstetrics that has been slow to change is the national rather than international orientation of the obstetrical (research) community. Dutch obstetricians still publish a considerable amount of their research in Dutch. For example, it was only after 1956 that dissertations started to be written in English, and until recently only 30 percent of all dissertations appeared in English. That such orientation to a local audience can be very disadvantageous became apparent in the 1960s, when two Dutch obstetricians missed international acknowledgment of the primacy of their research on amniocentesis because it had been published in Dutch.

In its ideals also, Dutch obstetrics shows a very constant picture with respect to its self-image as well as its views on pregnancy and delivery. Treub, the nineteenth-century professor of obstetrics in Amsterdam, fulfilled an exemplary role in this respect. The centenary of his birth was proudly celebrated by the association in 1956, and his name is still often connected to memorial events. Treub is admired partly because of the important work he has done for the association, including his efforts to build up a program of education and training in obstetrics, partly because of his early recognition of problems that in later years gained more and more prominence (contraception and abortion), and partly because of his personality. He had enlightened views on controversial matters, such as abortion and contraception, as well as on the moral and social position of women. He did not fear confrontations with the authorities, but publicly argued the need for additional provisions on the basis of his practice in Amsterdam. Generally, Treub is seen by obstetricians as the man who laid the foundations for obstetrics in the Netherlands. In these foundations, the conception that pregnancy is a physiological process is central, as is the idea that obstetricians should concentrate on the pathological cases. From the nineteenth century onwards, obstetricians in the Netherlands have pleaded for improvement and extension of the education of midwives, and for extension of their right to deal with normal pregnancies and deliveries.[32]

The Amsterdam clinic, important because of its size, profited from Treub's prominence as a teacher and public figure. This reputation has persisted up to the present. Just as Treub performed the first abortion for medical indications in the nineteenth century, even though it was illegal, so too Gerrit-Jan Kloosterman, Amsterdam professor from 1957 to 1982, performed the first abortions for other than strictly medical indications (equally against the law). Just as Treub had enlightened views on contraception, so too Kloosterman was the first obstetrician in the Netherlands to start a polyclinic for birth regulation. Just as Treub published the first Dutch textbook of obstetrics and gynecology in 1892, so in the 1970s Kloosterman took up the editorship of the textbook now used in all Dutch university departments.[33]

It is Kloosterman to whom the special reputation of the Amsterdam clinic in recent times is due, and whose name is often identified with a particular approach to pregnancy and delivery for which the Netherlands is so famous. In this approach, which is not limited to Amsterdam but has been most clearly developed and promoted there, we find concepts and ideas that have dominated Dutch obstetrics since the nineteenth century. It is characterized by an emphasis on the normal, nonclinical character of pregnancy and, according to Kloosterman's successor in Amsterdam, Professor P. E. Treffers, "a critical and relativizing attitude towards new therapies and widely announced medical achievements."[34] Medicalization of pregnancy and delivery is seen as an unwanted development; anesthesia and Caesarean section are avoided as much as possible; and home deliveries supervised by well-trained midwives are considered the ideal in normal circumstances. In the Dutch obstetrics textbook, edited by Kloosterman but a joint effort of all the obstetrics departments in the Netherlands, Kloosterman puts it as follows:

> A form of organization (of obstetric care) in which everyone is forced to go to hospital for the delivery as in the United States, seems first to have put at the center the interests and preferences of doctors. The segregation of healthy future mothers at home ... has a number of advantages: it underscores the physiological character of the event and stimulates the self-consciousness and self-reliance of the woman in labor; the cosy and home-like nature of her environment, to which her husband also has total access, works in the same direction.[35]

It is striking to find the mood here similar to the circles of the nineteenth-century NGV obstetricians as expressed in this quotation: coziness and a home-like atmosphere are highly valued elements, even in matters as serious as medicine. In the Amsterdam philosophy, a great deal of effort is put into strengthening first-line obstetric care and maintaining a high (academic) level of patient care. Education of obstetricians and future general practitioners (who still perform a substantial, although declining number of deliveries in the Netherlands) is a main point of attention. From a recent analysis of the Amsterdam obstetrics department, we learn that this emphasis has resulted in research oriented to evaluations of intra- and extramural obstetric care in which the social effects of the treatment were explicitly made part of the research question, as well as in laboratory research performed on patient materials (such as placentae) and animals. In this way, experimentation on women who are pregnant or in labor is kept to a minimum.[36] Furthermore, research aimed at preventing or predicting pathologies has naturally received much attention, for example, the construction of fetal growth curves. Papers are to a large extent directed at maintaining and strengthening the expertise of specialists, general practitioners, and midwives, and are published in Dutch medical periodicals.[37]

Although in more recent times conflicts and differences of opinion among obstetricians have been quite fierce, the striking thing about the Dutch situation is the relative absence of disagreements between the different parties involved. Women in the Netherlands have always appreciated the possibilities offered to them and have not seen any need to argue for the introduction of anesthesia or against routine episiotomy and high rates of Caesarean sections (as in the United States), or a high rate of inductions (as in Great Britain): these interventions in the normal course of the birth process have always been restricted to a minimum in the Netherlands.[38]

Midwives have profited from the protection they have had from obstetricians who have traditionally striven for improvements and extension of midwife training and education, while the boundaries of their practice have been extended (even in recent times) to include all "physiological pregnancies and deliveries" and the management of some special treatments, like episiotomies. As an indication of their status, it is interesting to note that in the 1979 law regulating midwives' authority, the title *vroedvrouw* (midwife) was replaced by *verloskundige*, which is the Dutch translation of obstetrician! In the Netherlands, the unique situation that has evolved resulted in midwives being called "experts in obstetrics," while in everyday language, obstetricians are usually referred to as gynecologists.

Finally, the Dutch state has given preference to home deliveries over routine hospital ones by reimbursing only the costs of a home delivery under the national health insurance (private insurers have also followed this policy) and by providing for a structure in which every woman is entitled to the help of a maternity home-care assistant who takes care of mother and baby and the household for eight (formerly ten) days after the delivery.

In Dutch obstetrics, quite a number of elements, already in evidence in the nineteenth century, have remained. These elements contribute to the special situation compared to other countries. Further, these elements have been paralleled by similarly special circumstances in the wider practice surrounding pregnancy and delivery. It is the interlocking of views and interests of the various parties involved that have been an important element in maintaining the structure as it is, and that have allowed for what has become the hallmark of the Dutch situation: the relatively large number of home deliveries.

The question now is whether this situation can withstand the pressures that drive it in the direction of something more in line with that of other modern Western countries. Several elements of the interlocking network of interests and views are changing. In fact, they have been changing slowly from

1960 onwards, when some 70 percent of the Dutch women had a home delivery, compared to some 36 percent now.

The character of the Dutch community of obstetricians has already started to change. In 1956 a fifth department of Obstetrics and Gynecology was established in a new university, and in the course of the following decade, three others followed. The number of departments and the number of student places doubled, while the number of professors quadrupled. The rising number of members of the NGV reflects this development: from 250 in 1962 to 650 in 1987. The growth has had implications beyond mere numbers of students and teachers, however, and the community of obstetricians began to lose its convivial character. No longer were all obstericians taught by the same people, leading to differing opinions and competition within the profession; moreover, the appointment of separate professors for obstetrics and gynecology resulted in further specialization.

In the universities, the last revision of the specialist licensing for obstetricians in 1961 secured the training for future specialists, and research became more and more important. There was a growing awareness of the disadvantages of publications restricted to a small linguistic area and the need to establish an international audience for research results. The editors of the *Nederlands Tijdschrift voor Verloskunde en Gynaecologie* regretfully saw many interesting articles offered to foreign (English language) journals.[39] In 1970, after many years of discussion, it was decided to strip the journal of its exclusively Dutch character and to proceed in English as the *European Journal of Obstetrics, Gynecology and Reproductive Biology*. This decision by the NGV to change its journal reflected the wish to become more international, but it was accompanied by words of sorrow and grief in the last issue of the *Nederlands Tijdschrift voor Verloskunde en Gynaecologie*. Other factors worked in the same direction: a rather unfavorable assessment of the obstetrics departments in a general evaluation of medical research achievements in the Netherlands, and a changing system of financing of university research.[40] This is a general trend, even in the stronghold of the Kloosterman school, the Amsterdam University Clinic; there is a growing emphasis on empirical research, and the younger members of staff have often been appointed expressly to stengthen this aspect.

Ideals have also changed. One of the newer departments of obstetrics has developed an approach to pregnancy and delivery very comparable to that in other countries.[41] The more international orientation of obstetricians has made Dutch obstetrics more vulnerable to the critical eye of its foreign colleagues, and critics from within the country have drawn support from that. They plead for hospital confinement for every primiparous woman and routine technological surveillance of the delivery process. Although it seems as if the situation has more or less stabilized now, in the 1960s and 1970s, the differences of opinion between the Amsterdam school and the more "hospital oriented" obstetricians led to very fierce debates.

Women themselves have increasingly opted to have delivery take place in the hospital. This was especially so when it became possible to give birth in the hospital and then return home within twenty-four hours without consequences for the availability of a home-care assistant.

Midwives as a group are doing well, although their position is still dependent on the protection of obstetricians. They have successfully competed with general practitioners over the supervision of home deliveries and are firmly established as a professional group,[42] but their practice is changing as well. Some midwives now prefer a hospital appointment, where working hours are regular and fixed. They have their practices in the hospital where they can make use of modern technology in the management of labor. Midwives in private practice are also beginning to acquire such technology (e.g., an ultrasound machine) in order to keep up with the fruits of clinical science that the hospital has to offer. Recently, midwives have been trying to develop a program of research in their own field: a trend towards scientification similar to other health-care fields, like nursing and physiotherapy. No doubt the scientification and academization of midwives' practices will have profound effects on the structure and content of the profession. Finally, the Dutch state has also contributed to the changes since the 1960s by allowing for reimbursement of the twenty-four-hour hospital delivery in the national health insurance scheme.

So, although the home deliveries, the hallmark of Dutch obstetric practice, now amount to some 35 percent of all deliveries in the Netherlands, the question is whether this will remain the case. How has this practice been able to withstand the onslaught of scientific medicine for so long, and will it continue to do so now, when the foundations on which it is based seem to be changing? Of course this is a complex question that requires further study. From the few studies that have been done, it is clear that various processes and forces at different points in time have been important. For example, in the state support for home deliveries, economic considerations have played a role along with ideological ones, and competition between gynecologists and general practitioners has to some extent motivated the former's support for midwives. Nevertheless, these are general factors, and do not explain the typical and unique Dutch situation. Part of the explanation may well have to take into account the special position the family has always had in Dutch society. The nuclear family provided the place for such an intimate and private event as the birth of a baby, and violation of such privacy by outsiders was kept to a minimum.[43] The anonymity of the hospital and of the specialist doctor was seen as a necessity only in emergencies, and the specialists refrained as much as possible from intervening in the pregnancies of the patients in the hospital. The central role of the Dutch family has been crucial: it follows that the significance of the nuclear family during childbirth in the Netherlands requires cultural explanation. The relationship between women and midwife-friendly obstetrics even now derives from widely shared cultural values about the meaning and place of pregnancy and delivery. In the rather protected cultural environment of Dutch society, such values may have been responsible for the consensus from groups with different interests. In this view, the birth of a baby is a fundamentally natural and therefore sacred process that should not be interfered with, and women who are delivering a child should be well aware and grateful for this special privilege. In such a view, giving anesthesia for labor pains is similar to depriving a woman of a valuable and deeply personal experience; any unnecessary interference is seen as an unwanted arrogance of doctors who think they can do better than nature. The importance of shared cosmologies was recognized by Kloosterman:

> The recognition that it is not only rational scientific arguments that are hidden behind the various systems of organization [of obstetric care], but even more so emotional, cosmological arguments that mostly remain unconscious and therefore give extra vigor to (pseudo) scientific arguments, that is the necessary condition to understand why such fierce and personal debates are being held precisely about the obstetrical organization.[44]

The breakdown of these values since the end of the 1960s has made for a situation in which the different participants cannot so easily find common ground to reach a consensus. This may be the greatest threat to the unique character of Dutch obstetric science and practice. Because of this fundamental and growing uncertainty, the developments of the last twenty years may now result in unwarranted and profound changes of the field of obstetrics in the Netherlands. In my opinion, that would be a great loss.

NOTES

This chapter is revised from an article titled "Obstetrics Research in the Netherlands in the Nineteenth Century," in *Medical History* 31 (1987): 281–305, copyright the Trustees of the Wellcome Trust, and is produced with their permission. Many of the references in Dutch have been omitted from this version.

1. For a thorough political-economic history of the Netherlands and Belgium, *see* Kossmann, E. H., *The Low Countries, 1780–1940* (Oxford: Clarendon Press, 1978).

2. Ibid., p. 137.

3. Ibid., p. 179.

4. Many writers have indicated these factors as important characteristics of the process of professionalization. *See*, for example, Friedson, E., *Profession of Medicine: A Study of the Sociology of Applied Knowledge* (New York: Dodd, Mead, 1970); Johnson, T., *Professions and Power* (London: Macmillan, 1972).

5. Ackerknecht, E. H., *A Short History of Medicine* (Baltimore: Johns Hopkins University Press, 1968).

6. Van Geuns, J., *De Geneeskunde als Zelfstandige Wetenschap*, inaugural lecture held in Amsterdam, January 28, 1847, pp. 2–3.

7. Ackerknecht, *A Short History*; Geison, G. L., "Divided we stand: physiologists and clinicians in the American context," in *The Therapeutic Revolution*, Vogel, J., and C. E. Rosenberg (eds.) (Philadelphia: University of Pennsylvania Press, 1979): 67–91.

8. Minutes of the meeting of the clinical school professors, June 21, 1858, Amsterdam, Municipal Archive, File 30 nr. 25.

9. Lehmann, L., *Het Tegenwoordige Standpunt der Geneeskunde met Hare Licht en Schaduwzijde* (Amsterdam, 1870): 4.

10. Ibid., p. 13.

11. Ibid., p. 8.

12. Mendelsohn, E., "The Social Construction of Scientific Knowledge," in *The Social Production of Scientific Knowledge*, Mendelsohn, E., and P. Weingart (eds.) (Dordrecht: Reidel, 1977); Weindling, "Theories of the Cell State in Imperial Germany," in *Biology, Medicine and Society, 1840–1940* Webster, C., (ed.) (Cambridge: Cambridge University Press, 1981): 99–157, particularly stress this "double" engagement of the German progressive doctors.

13. Opening lecture of Professor C. A. Pekelharing of the NMG, July 2, 1888, published in *NTG* 1888.

14. This seems to have been the case much longer. D. de Moulin (*Janus* 45 (1978): 21-44) describes this orientation and the importation of German doctors as something already apparent in the seventeenth century. The Germans were present not only as practicing doctors and university teachers, they also sat on editorial boards of medical journals and practiced as military doctors.

15. This legislation dates from August 8, 1822. No foreigners were allowed to be appointed professor unless they were naturalized.

16. See Cooter, R., "Anticontagionism and History's Medical Record," in *The Problem of Medical Knowledge*, Wright, P. and A. Treacher (eds.) (Edinburgh: Edinburgh University Press, 1982) about the relationship between medicine and ideology in the case of anticontagionism. For a more thorough and interesting account, one should read E. H. Ackerknecht, "Anticontagionism between 1821 and 1867," *Bulletin of the History of Medicine* 22 (1948): 562–593.

17. C. A. Pekelharing in his opening lecture to the NMG, published in *NTG* 2:7 (1888). In 1891 Treub proposed to separate education again into a practically and a scientifically oriented direction, although not with the same differences in licensing as before the 1865 law. He thought to do this by reducing the number of universities from four to two and by turning the other two into medical schools.

18. Professor C. M. Kan cited these statements from the *Municipal Journal* in his speech to the University of Amsterdam staff and students on the occasion of handing over the rectorship in 1893.

19. G. C. Nijhoff wrote this in one of his regular reviews of dissertations in obstetrics in *NTvVG* (1889), p. 248.

20. Treub, H., *De Gevaren der Hedendaagse Gynecologie* (Leiden, 1896): 385.

21. In an editorial announcement in *Weekblad van het Nederlandsch Tijdschrift voor Geneeskunde* 1: 18 (1897): 701.

22. Quoted by B. J. Kouwer in the introduction to the register of the index of *NTvVG* (1931), p. 15, from the minutes of the Dutch Gynecological Association (NGV).

23. Yearly report of the NGV, published in *NTvVG* (1897), pp. 321–323.

24. Kouwer, see note 22 above, p. 31.

25. Ibid., p. 21.

26. Simmer, H. H., "Principles and problems of medical undergraduate education in Germany during the nineteenth and early twentieth centuries," in *The History of*

Medical Education, O'Malley, C. D. (ed.), UCLA Forum Medical Science no. 12 (Los Angeles: University of California Press, 1970): 173–200, especially p. 187 on.

27. Turner, S. S., "The growth of professional research in Prussia, 1818 to 1848—causes and context," *Historical Studies in the Physical Sciences* 3 (1971): 137–182.

28. Sometimes this point is stressed by reference to the relative number of scientific discoveries in nineteenth-century German medicine, as is done by Ben-David, J., "Scientific productivity and academic organization in nineteenth-century medicine," *American Sociological Review* 35 (1960): 828–843; Zloczower, A., *Career Opportunities and the Growth of Scientific Discovery in Nineteenth-Century Germany* (New York: Arno Press, 1981).

29. Flexner, A., *Medical Education in Europe* (New York: Carnegie Foundation Bulletin no. 6, 1912). See also Ben-David and Zloczower cited in note 28. This point is also made in the introduction to Lemaine, G. et al., *Perspectives on the Emergence of Scientific Disciplines* (The Hague: Mouton, 1976): 7.

30. In 1956, in the new (Catholic) University of Nijmegen, a chair of obstetrics and gynecology was created. In Amsterdam, a second university was founded (on Dutch Reformed religious principles) where a chair of obstetrics and gynecology was established in 1962. In the new universities of Rotterdam and Maastricht, chairs of obstetrics and gynecology were created in 1967 and 1978, respectively. Only in the course of the 1970s were separate chairs of obstetrics and gynecology established in all Dutch universities.

31. The proportion of deliveries attended by general practitioners fell from 46 percent in 1960 to 26 percent in 1973 and 16 percent in 1986.

32. The first report of Dutch obstetricians on the education of midwives dates from 1897. At the request of the NMG, a committee of the NGV was installed to advise on how the level of education and the position of midwives could be improved. Based on an inquiry among doctors, an overwhelming majority of whom supported midwives, the committee advised strengthening the position of midwives by creating a more rigorous selection process and by recruiting women from the middle classes; by a longer and more scientifically oriented program of education and training; by establishing a special journal for midwives; and by trying to prevent competition among midwives and general practitioners by forbidding doctors from taking a smaller fee for a delivery than midwives. This report set the tone for future advice on these matters from the obstetricians. It was published in the *NTG* 1 (1897), p. 610. Other committees were established in 1911, 1952, and 1979, leading to the extension of midwives' education from two to three years and to extensions of their authority in 1979 to include "all physiological deliveries."

33. Kloosterman, G. J. (ed.), *De Voortplanting van de Mens: Leerboek voor Obstetrie en Gynecologie* (Bussum: Centen, 1973). This textbook is a common enterprise of ten (later eleven) universities, including all departments of obstetrics and gynecology. In the foreword, it is stated that the text was intended for a Dutch audience because of the special situation in this field in the Netherlands.

34. In the *Liber Amicorum* offered to Kloosterman at the occasion of his twenty-five-year professorship in Amsterdam, the Kloosterman approach is characterized by the following elements: respect for and curiosity in the physiology of pregnancy and delivery; careful quantitative approach to obstetric problems (for example, the study

of growth curves of fetuses); the influence of placental weight and infarction on birth weight and perinatal mortality; very careful indications with respect to gynecological therapeutic management and an absence of easy operative interference; interest in psychological aspects of obstetrics.

35. Kloosterman's textbook, see note 33 above. Page 390 in the 1981 and later editions.

36. Prins, A.A.M., and K. Boekhorst, *De Praktijk van het Patientgebonden Onderzoek*, Report published by the Department of Science Dynamics, Amsterdam, 1987, pp. 62–63.

37. Ibid., pp. 83–86.

38. For descriptions and analyses of the situation in the United States and Great Britain, see Wertz, Richard W., and Dorothy C. Wertz, *Lying-In: A History of Childbirth in America* (New York: The Free Press, 1979); Leavitt, J. Waltzer, *Brought to Bed: Childbearing in America, 1750–1950* (New York: Oxford, 1986); Leavitt, J. W., and W. Walton, "Down to death's door: women's perception of childbirth in America," in *Women and Health in America*, Leavitt, J. Waltzer (ed.) (Madison/London, 1984): 155–166; Arney, W. R., *Power and the Profession of Obstetrics* (Chicago: University of Chicago Press, 1982); Oakley, A., *The Captured Womb: A History of the Medical Care of Pregnant Women* (Oxford: Basil Blackwell, 1984).

39. In the editorial of the first issue of the *European Journal of Obstetrics and Gynecology*, the initiative was motivated in the following way: "to create a journal that, although published by both societies [the Belgian and Dutch Societies for Obstetrics and Gynecology A. H.] primarily intends to serve as a rostrum for all clinicians and investigators in Europe and abroad who want their work to be known in a wider field than enclosed in historical boundaries" (1971), p. 1.

40. Blume, S. S. and J. B. Spaapen, "External assessment and conditional financing of research in Dutch universities," *Minerva* 26 (1988): 1–30.

41. The main representatives of this approach can be found in the relatively young Department of Obstetrics and Gynecology of the Catholic University of Nijmegen, led by Professor K.A.B. Eskes.

42. See van Daalen, R., "Dutch obstetric care: home or hospital, midwife or gynecologist," *Health Prom.* 2:3 (1988): 247–255.

43. In line with this conception of the nuclear family is the position of the general practitioner in the Netherlands. The general practitioner has traditionally been very close to the family; he would know the parents, grandparents, and children of his patients; he would come to the house if someone were ill, and would pay interested visits on his own initiative to older patients or patients in hospital to see how they were doing. As a family doctor, he would be available twenty-four hours a day, and patients would also consult him for nonmedical problems. It is not surprising that such a paternalistic role was performed almost exclusively by men. Although the close arrangement has loosened somewhat in recent times, the Dutch general practitioner is still a family doctor and pays home visits when patients are unable to come to his office. Furthermore, he is the main source of referrals to specialists, because all types of health insurances require a referral note from a general practitioner before reimbursement for specialist care.

44. Kloosterman, J. G., "Zwangerschapskunde," in Boer, K. and H. Chamalaun (eds.), *Over Voortplanting Gesproken* (Groningen: Wolters Noordhof, 1985): 93.

4

Family Change and Continuity in the Netherlands: Birth and Childbed in Text and Art

Rineke van Daalen

When a baby is born, Dutch parents prefer their own domestic surroundings. About 70 percent of the mothers of newborn children stay at home during childbed. Half of them also give birth at home; half of them choose a short stay in the hospital.[1] For all, well-organized maternity home care is readily available. This emphasis on domesticity was an important part of the background to the continuous existence of home delivery; it also slowed down the pace of medicalization. Only with the introduction of the short-stay hospital birth in 1965, with its possibility of going home as soon as possible, did hospital delivery begin to find acceptance in the Netherlands. The popularity of the short-stay clinical delivery was and still is related to the combination of security offered by a hospital and the *gezelligheid*, or reassurance of the home environment.[2] The strong emphasis on the home environment for birth and childbed is one of the features that makes the Dutch obstetric pattern exceptional in the Western world. This pattern is associated with a relatively low degree of medicalization and an important and autonomous role for the midwives who assist the woman during pregnancy and birth. Along with the conception of birth as a natural process is the tendency to limit the amount of medical interventions.

In addition, what makes the specific character of contemporary Dutch patterns of pregnancy, birth, and childbed so unique can also be located in the history of the Dutch family from the seventeenth century onward. The first section of this chapter treats the rise of domesticity in Dutch family life from the aspects of common lore and social science. The second section includes a historical-sociological study of Dutch birth and childbed in the seventeenth

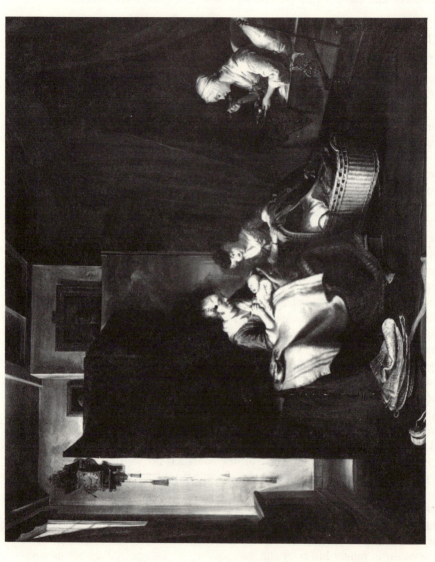

Cornelis Troos, "De Hollandse Kraamkamer" ("Dutch Childbed Scene"), 1737. Museum Boymans-vab Beuningen, Rotterdam. Publication: *Successful Home Birth and Midwifery.*

and early eighteenth centuries. This section rests on a range of primary sources, from pictures to plays and treatises by doctors and midwives. The conclusion deals with the relation between the development of the Dutch family, especially its nuclearization and privatization concerning birth and childbed, and the exceptional obstetric system of the Netherlands.

THE NUCLEARIZATION AND DOMESTICATION OF WESTERN FAMILY LIFE

One of the important changes in family life in the modern period is the rise of the conjugal family and its withdrawal from the community. Philippe Ariès, Edward Shorter, Lawrence Stone, and Jean-Louis Flandrin, whose work has been characterized by Michael Anderson as the "sentiments approach," argued that in the sixteenth century the notion of an independent nuclear family was absent from almost all sections of the population. Individuals and households were embedded in the wider community; they had important nonfamily relationships and a strong sense of communality. What is known as gemeinschaftliche[3] family relations gradually moved towards increasing individualism and differentiation of the conjugal family as a discrete, private, and venerated social unit with an emphasis on domesticity.[4] The next generation of historians of family life, the revisionists, claimed that early family historians exaggerated the differences between premodern and modern societies, especially the hypotheses relating to changes in sentiments between parents and their children as well as between lovers and spouses.[5] There is general agreement among sociologists and social historians, however, about the gradual nuclearization of families, the separation of family relations from the wider community, and the privatization of families. They see indications for this increasing privacy in the disappearance of outsiders from the smaller households and in the rise of a "closed" and spatially divided domestic architecture. Consensus exists as well about the diminishing interference and concern of the community in family life. In modern societies, it does not play an important role in spouse selection, childbirth and death, and organized public rituals at marriages; nor do institutionalized public demonstrations of community control, such as charivaris, exist to discipline and punish the adulterous and the lewd.

We believe that relations between family and community and intercourse within the family are historical variables. This chapter concentrates on the nuclearization and domestication of family relations in the Netherlands,[6] particularly the timing and degree of those processes. The most important controversies in family history relate particularly to the chronology of changes, the regions where the changes occurred, the sequence in which different social groups enacted these changes, and above all, the causes of change. Specialized studies, like this one on seventeenth-century Netherlands, contribute to a better understanding of these changes and how they occurred in one part of Europe while giving us a broader comprehension of family history in general.

The privatization and seclusion of family life were parts of a more general process of civilization that involved changes in behavior and mentalities and a broad range of intimate and physical human activities. When births take place, for example, the community has become less significant.

Where nuclearization of family life took place, it was accompanied by a division of tasks between men working for money and women doing household work and looking after husband and children. Motherly care, also for infants and toddlers, became a virtue and an ideal. The associated improvements in mothering formed, in combination with an increasing domesticity, the core of the genesis of the nuclear family.[7] These developments may be seen as different aspects of a disintegration of preindustrial, small-scale community life, as a transition of long duration from *Gemeinschaft* to *Gesellschaft*. During this process, secular elites were withdrawing from popular cultures, and several separate cultures came into being, from court and town cultures to more traditional ones.

DUTCH DOMESTICITY

As early as the seventeenth and eighteenth centuries, people were struck by certain characteristics of Dutch families. The observations of foreign visitors and some Dutch observers were similar in two respects: the Dutch had a stronger attachment to hearth and home and, along with this, their family life had an inward, withdrawn character, with little public interventions. The devoted care to furnishings and maintenance of domestic surroundings attested to the value placed on interior domestic scenes. This special attention to the interior of the house went together with the proverbial cleanliness and neatness of Dutch women, which seemed amazing to foreign visitors. Dutch women would idolize their houses and furniture, while neglecting other issues. They did not restrict their activities to the interior of their home, but even swept and scrubbed the streets that gave access to it. In *The Embarrassment of Riches*, Simon Schama quotes a series of foreigners about the tidiness of Dutch housewives, while he himself points out the moral character of Dutch purity rituals.[8]

A number of authors, Dutch and foreign, writing in different periods see a relationship between the cult of the home and the tendency towards domestic family life. They portray the seventeenth-century Dutch as people who spent most of their time in their own houses, originating in the need for cozy warmth and intimacy. They would only make small visits to friends and relatives and short business tours to neighboring towns. In spite of their thrift, domesticity caused them to spend enormous amounts of money and energy in decorating and cleaning their houses. Foreigners were amazed not only by

Dutch domestic life, but also by the loving relations between Dutch spouses and between parents and children.

Opinions about Dutch domestic culture and family life are based on generally held ideas. Whether such assertions about the social history of Dutch family life are true can be tested through historical and sociological research.

A study of marriage and family in Holland in the seventeenth and eighteenth centuries gives supporting evidence. Various sources—correspondences, treatises of moralists, documents of legal proceedings, inquiries into the paternity of illegitimate children—provided the information for the development of a specific Dutch constellation. Compared with families from other European countries, Dutch family members did have more egalitarian relations. Moreover, the nuclear family was relatively independent and privately oriented.[9] This last point accords with the observations of seventeenth-century fellow countrymen and foreigners about Dutch domestic family life.

The close family orientation and individualistic attitude are reflected in the architectural practices of seventeenth-century Amsterdam householders. In the grander houses, residence was separated from business, and the Amsterdam burgher did not wish this residence subordinated to a comprehensive whole: the identity of individual houses was never submerged into a larger architectural composition, as was the case in seventeenth- and eighteenth-century London and Paris. The leading successful merchant families used a portion of their profits for domestic display, for homes with more assertive pomp than the houses of London merchants. A comparison between the social history of Venetian and Amsterdam elites from about 1580 to about 1720 gives a somewhat different impression. Houses of the Amsterdam elite were more modest than in Venice and do not seem to have had the symbolic importance of the Venetian palaces. "The works of architecture and sculpture commissioned by the Amsterdam élite show ... less magnificence, less display and less desire for the conspicuous glorification of the family."[10] The Amsterdam houses were above all places for the nuclear family to live in. In that respect, the Amsterdam *burghers* excelled. They paid much attention to the furnishing and decoration of the interior of their houses, which is another indication of the value they attached to domesticity. The exterior simplicity contrasted with interior splendor, but both focused on showing off to the world outside.

The domestic and private character of Dutch family life is not only a phenomenon from the past. In a sociological study about the Netherlands in the 1960s, Johan Goudsblom points to the shared impression that the Dutch would cherish the private rather than the public sphere and that they would seek comfort first in the family. This common impression is supported by official figures: until the radical changes in family life in the 1960s, the Dutch went less often to cafes or movie theaters than people in neighboring countries. Family culture and family cohesion were highly valued, which Goudsblom sees related to the *burgher* inheritance.[11] *Burghers* predominated in the *Republic*, which was not a dynastic state or an extended polis. It was governed by urban upper strata, especially *burghers*, patricians, and merchants.[12]

Another starting point for understanding the domestic tendency of the Dutch may be found in the important place of the Calvinist religion in the Netherlands. Among Calvinists, the nuclear family was held in high esteem. Husband and wife should have an affectionate relationship, and parents should account to God for the education of their children.

According to Donald Haks (1985), the privatization of the nuclear family in the Netherlands took place earlier, contacts with neighbors were less obliging, and social control was less penetrating than in other parts of western Europe. Spouse selection and, to a lesser degree, divorce were primarily left to the persons concerned. The conjugal family was the dominant family type in seventeenth- and eighteenth-century Holland.[13] In the upper social strata, especially among urban *burghers*, the rise of an autonomous family life implied above all independence from broader networks of relatives. In those small elite nuclear families, the origin of domesticity and intimacy must be found. Parents spent much time and energy on the education of their children, who were growing up in small households, without relatives and without many servants.[14]

Assertions about the Dutch inclination to domesticity and the seclusion of family life are common lore, and have been confirmed in the recent work of social historians and sociologists. Do these observations also apply to pregnancy, birth, and childbed in the Netherlands? We believe that in the Netherlands, the privatization of birth and childbed came about earlier, and the changes that went with it were more sweeping than elsewhere in western Europe.

THE PRIVATIZATION OF BIRTH AND CHILDBED IN THE NETHERLANDS

The process of privatization of births has a long history in Western societies. During the Middle Ages and in the sixteenth and seventeenth centuries, births were not surrounded by extreme secrecy or absolute privacy.[15] Women had their babies in the presence of people from the community.[16]

In the Netherlands, there was an emphasis on domesticity and intimate family life in connection with processes of privatization of birth. In the nineteenth and twentieth centuries, champions of home birth used this emphasis to argue against clinical births. In 1826, for example, the Rotterdam municipality stated that institutional births and maternity wards would not fit Dutch society and would be incompatible with the Dutch "national character." Women in labor, including the poor, would not only object to being used as objects for educational ends, they would also be opposed to a separation from their relatives.[17] Furthermore, 140 years later, the well-known obstetrician Kloosterman (chapter 11) followed a comparable line of reasoning in defense of Dutch home birth, which he saw as pre-eminently appropriate to the Dutch population. These statements illustrate the Dutch preference for home birth and the need to be among relatives or friends during labor. Together, the statements describe a privatized context of birth, spatial and social, which differs not only from the isolation of modern medicalized birth, but also from the image we have of Western traditional births as community events, with many neighbors and relatives present and with inquisitive crowds outside.

Edward Shorter mentions some eighteenth-century examples of such social events, one in Boston with eight women present in the lying-in room, and one in France with more than thirty women present.[18] A comparably crowded birth in 1878 in Sappemeer, a small village in the north of the Netherlands, has been sketched by Aletta Jacobs, the first Dutch female doctor and one of the first feminists. She describes how she came upon a large company of relatives, friends, and neighbors, all smoking and drinking in the same room as the laboring woman, giving advice and help.[19] We may infer from Jacobs' description that the views expressed by the Rotterdam governors as well as Kloosterman do not describe nineteenth-century births in the Dutch countryside. Jacobs' experience and Shorter's examples indicate that home birth did not always go together with privacy. In traditional societies, neighbors did have a regular role in important family events, like childbirth. Home births as intimate events within a small group were characteristic for nuclear families. The processes of privatization took place a long time before the medicalization and the hospitalization of birth. The timing of these processes in the Netherlands seems to have been out of step compared with other European countries: the privatization of the nuclear family seems to have evolved earlier, and the medicalization of birth took place later than elsewhere in the Western world.

Both processes are peculiarly urban phenomena.[20] This is crucial to bear in mind when comparing the social history of Dutch family relations with that of other countries. In the Netherlands, processes of urbanization had made early progress, especially in the province of Holland, where in 1514 about 46 percent of the population was living in towns, in 1622 54 percent, and in 1795 59 percent. The distance between villages and towns was not very large, and the roads were quite good for that period.[21] This urbanized character of the country may have contributed to an early nuclearization of family relations.

DUTCH PREGNANCY, BIRTH, AND CHILDBED IN TEXTS

Special regulations for women in childbed were already in effect in the first half of the fifteenth century in the Netherlands and Germany. Their houses (*kraamhuizen*) were seen as holy and were declared inviolable, by decree and on pain of a fine. Those who were pursued could even seek sanctuary in such houses. Legal regulations of this type were issued by, for example, Count Karel de Stoute and the Duke of Gelderlandt.[22] Originally, these regulations were associated with the supernatural, but later they were gradually enlarged and secularized. It was felt that a family having a baby should be respected; noise should be kept to a minimum in and around a *kraamhuis*, and the father and his friends should not be allowed to celebrate birth in a boisterous way. Creditors should suspend their claims during childbed, writs against the family could not be issued, and those who checked the weight of bread, for example, should spare families with a newborn baby. Passers-by were warned by cloth wrappings around the bell and the latch of the front door of a *kraamhuis*.[23]

The regulations designed to ensure the peace of those in childbed changed during the sixteenth and seventeenth centuries. The arguments in favor of protection and privatization of the *kraamhuis* turned from sacral to secular. In the earlier ordinances from the fifteenth and sixteenth centuries, the focus was primarily directed towards the sacred character of the events around birth and towards the guarantee of immunity for all persons involved. Later, in the seventeenth and eighteenth centuries, the peace and need for rest of the mother and child were used as arguments for protection. On the streets in front of the house, sand and straw were sprinkled to deaden the noise of carriages passing by. The latch of the door of a *kraamhuis* was no longer covered in cloth; instead, a refined fan-like decoration was placed there, a *kloppertje*, different for boys and girls. People who wanted to inquire after the health of mother and child were received by a maid-servant in the entrance hall, or they could read a small letter describing the birth and the health of mother and child placed in the window.

In the eighteenth century, an even more distant way of announcing births was introduced among people of high standing who lived in towns. They ordered an undertaker's assistant to pass the news to acquaintances nearby, and they sent printed messages to acquaintances living farther away. In the same period, the traditional custom of collective visits by neighbors was replaced by more individual childbed visits in the upper classes. Visitors came in small numbers, one by one.

Not only was the house protected against the world outside, but inside the house a special room, the *kraamkamer*, was furnished and decorated for the lying-in period, in accordance with fixed, almost ritual patterns. The old-Dutch carefulness was especially apparent in preparations for an oncoming birth. This seventeenth- and eighteenth-century upper-class custom of setting up a *kraamkamer* was, according to some authors, typically Dutch,[24] although the true origin of such rooms was among the fifteenth-century Spanish and French monarchs and aristocracy.[25] For the seventeenth-century Dutch and the fifteenth-century French and Spanish aristocracy, *kraamkamers* functioned as occasions for display to the outer world. Just as with mourning, the *kraamkamers* expressed the pomp and hierarchical distinctions. They confirmed the existing social hierarchy. The interior of the *kraamkamers*, with their special furniture for the woman in labor, for the baby, and for the dry nurse, and with their special objects, such as the *bakermat* (a rush basket for the dry nurse), the *kraamscherm* (the special lying-in screen for protecting mother and child against drafts and the curious), the baby-linen basket, the baby clothes, the blankets, the cradle, and the pincushion, all expressed the social status of the family and at the same time showed the care and competence of the mother. Arranging a *kraamkamer* was both a family affair and a way of displaying one's social status and standing within the community. The mother-to-be was assisted by her mother-in-law or if she was absent, by her own mother. When preparations were finished, the pregnant woman invited neighbors and relatives for an inspection. Her arrangements accorded with the prosperity of the family, neither too ostentatious nor too poor, and demonstrated her motherly virtue. The *kraamkamers* were typical for the upper classes, but they do not seem to have been restricted to the elite. They could vary a great deal, from simple to very complicated.

In examining how birth was embedded in the community, it is important to know who and how many people were present, and the kind of activities they were involved in. An examination of the writings of midwives from the period provides a good picture. The midwives, like the dry nurses, were paid, occupational helpers; their time had to be reserved weeks before the baby was due. Neighbors were also called in. Kelderman, a man-midwife, wrote in 1697 in his instruction book for midwives that three or four women should be present in the *kraamkamer* in addition to the midwife to assist the woman in labor. For the neighbors help was a social obligation, and they had a well-defined task: three of them should support the women in labor and one should warm the infant's clothes.[26]

Writing in her journal about her work in the countryside of the province of Friesland, the midwife Catherina Schrader, who demonstrates an impressive expertise in obstetric issues, gives comparable but scant information about the presence of others at a birth. In the context of her notes, this subject is of secondary importance, but her oblique remarks make it clear that in her practice, neighbors did have a function at births.[27] Donald Haks also mentions the presence at a birth of four or five neighbors and relatives who lived in nearby towns; in the countryside, sometimes these women would come from neighboring villages. The neighbors gave assistance and support. Moreover, in case of an illegitimate birth, they were witnesses when the mother revealed the name of the father.

Changes in the festive celebrations after birth happened at different rates in the various social strata. Festivities in the countryside took a different course than those in the towns. In all social circles, the female neighbors were treated to a drink in the house of the childbed: the rich drank *kandeel*, the typical birth drink; the poor served a *kraam-anijsje*. The father invited his friends to the wine house, but the celebrations varied in degree of sobriety and privacy. Among farmers, the feasts were often exuberant and less moderate than among *burghers*. Peasant women, fathers, farmhands, and maids danced in the yard, and passers-by were forced to join them and give tips. If they were stiff, they were caught by the women, wrapped in a blanket and swaddled like a baby.

This kind of peasant scene was indeed a community event, just like the traditional births Shorter (1982) referred to. In the towns, it was somewhat different. A popular farce, *Kraam-bed of kandeel-maal van Zaartje Jans*, written in 1683, shows who would be present at the birth festivities in circles of the "petite bourgeoisie" in Amsterdam.[28] Naturally the play is fiction, but the women, who are only background characters for the comic and painful events that form the central theme of the story, have documentary value. The grandmother and the dry nurse have prepared the *kandeelmaal* and invited eight women from the neighborhood to participate. Although the father is present part of the time, the meal is a female affair. The women speak about the course of the delivery and the qualities of the midwife, they inquire after the mother's breasts, they praise the nursing, and they admire the baby. The gathering may be characterized as sober, but not stingy—the element of generosity towards outsiders is present. Although it is a social event, only a few invited guests are welcome.

People from the elite, aristocracy, and upper middle class took even greater pains to distance themselves from people outside the small family. They formed an avant-garde in protecting the childbed. They no longer participated in the sumptuous banquets that used to be given in honor of a newborn baby immediately following the birth, during the first childbed period, at baptism, and at the mother's first visit to church. From the fourteenth century onwards, bylaws (*keuren*) were passed to restrict these feasts and banquets, as they were for wedding parties and funeral meals. They were forbidden by the court (*'t Geregt*), as were restrictions on the number of visitors who were permitted and their demeanor. Although similar regulations were repeatedly enacted since the Middle Ages without much success, later restrictions were more effective. At the end of the eighteenth century, there were no longer any new bylaws enacted. From his description of the celebrations after childbirth, the historiographer J. Le Francq van Berkhey saw a distinction between the customs of the elite and those of the common people in the eighteenth century. The elite and townspeople celebrated the coming of a new baby in a more intimate circle than the common people. In this respect, they were distanced from popular culture, popular festivities, customs, and rituals, which they increasingly considered as vulgar.[29]

DUTCH CHILDBED IN ART

The representation of birth goes back to Italian religious art. In the cathedral of Siena, for example, religious images dating from the beginning of the fourteenth century showing the birth of Mary and of Christ have been portrayed on altarpieces; in the Santa Maria Novela in Florence, the birth of

Johannes has been depicted from the end of the fourteenth century. In the Netherlands, many pictures of childbed scenes of a secular character were made in the seventeenth and eighteenth centuries. From these works, we derive more insight into the socio-genesis of Dutch birth customs. The events in the *kraamkamer* just after birth have been a popular theme of Dutch genre artists.[30] Many painters from both the North and South were interested in those scenes, and they represented this intimate family episode, one that is now often photographed and even videotaped. Some painters, such as Anthonie Palamedesz (1601–73), Jan Horemans (1682–1759), and Cornelis Troost (1696–1750), did several series of *kraamkamers*, some of which were copied. Did Dutch painters in this period represent such scenes more often than painters from other Western countries?[31] The large amount of *kraamkamer* paintings is partly an artifact of the enormous volume of the total art production of Dutch painters in the Golden Age.[32] The possession of paintings was not reserved to an elite. In Amsterdam, the kinds of paintings of which the *kraamkamers* formed part, the genre pieces, ranked third in the order of preference, after landscapes and portraits. They were among the least expensive pictures, along with landscapes and still lifes. Together they accounted for about half of the total production of paintings in Holland in the Republic.[33]

The large number of childbed scenes must be understood within the general context of the production and consumption of genre pictures. During the seventeenth century, the diversity of themes in genre pieces was growing, along with an increasing interest in representations of indoor scenes of an intimate and sober character. The choice of *kraamkamers* as a subject for painting fits this tradition, as it also fits the Dutch tradition of representing scenes with elements derived from daily life, but this does not explain the tendency to depict *kraam* scenes in particular. Large domains of daily life were hardly ever pictured by seventeenth-century painters.[34] This was the case with birth and its immediate after-pains as physical events, scenes that were probably regarded as unbecoming.

Portrayals of childbed scenes were appropriate for a cultivated setting and, as appears from the large production, attractive in collector circles. They pictured the events after the quiet in the family had been restored. Anything that was disturbing and reminded people of the dangerous, physical, and sexual sides of birth was removed. All pictures show one room, containing a group of people gathered to honor the newborn child. Mother and child are present in every picture, but the rest of the company varies in number and composition. The position of mother and child varies as well. Sometimes the mother is lying in bed in the background; sometimes it is difficult to distinguish her from the other women. Sometimes the baby is the center of the activities: the adults are occupied with the care of the infant, or its social inauguration is at stake. At other times, the baby's position is subordinate.

The events have a festive character manifested in a decorative setting or in eating and drinking.

To what extent do the *kraamkamer* scenes refer to Dutch customs and experience in the seventeenth and eighteenth centuries, and to what extent do they have symbolic meanings? Do the images depict everyday events, or are they only the surface that reflects "a trend in the direction of a realistic disguise of allegories"?[35] If the world of pictures is an extension of the world of experience, is the former meant as an example, a fallacy, a terror, or a phantasm?[36] Apart from interpreting any inscriptions, signs, or symbols that appear in the pictures, reflecting on the social context in which pictures were produced and distributed is a way of relating art to the real world and recovering its signification.

It may be possible to discern the wishes and influence of the purchasers by researching their relation to the painters. In the seventeenth century, painters worked either on the basis of commissions from local governments, especially in big cities like Amsterdam, or on commissions from *burghers*, mostly merchants, as private persons, and as governors. Artists also sought buyers in a free market, especially for still lifes, landscapes, seascapes, and genre pieces. Their customers were middle-class people (shopkeepers, guildmasters, and merchants) who purchased paintings like furniture. The church did not commission many works, and the role of the court as patron is controversial.[37]

Apart from commissions and purchasers in the free market, there was a third category, the circle of wealthy collectors consisting of Dutch *burghers* and European aristocracy, who did not give special instructions to painters, but kept personal contact with them. Paintings for this group were rarely made for one special client, nor were they sold to anonymous buyers. It is more difficult to document intentions from this secular private art than from public and religious art, which was the product of patronage and often had a didactic tenor. The images represented ideals of civilization, both good and bad, that related to domestic life. They were intended to portray a virtuous and sensible life. *Kraamkamers* were not ordered by public institutions. The pictures of painter and actor Cornelis Troost were bought by the art-loving circle around him. Troost did at least ten *kraamkamers*.[38] He was living in Amsterdam among artists and intellectuals who admired his work. Among those who displayed his paintings and drawings was Jeronimus Tonneman, who financed Troost. Data from auction catalogs indicate that at least one early possessor of Troost's *kraamkamers* was a friend of his, while another was a son-in-law.[39] Because the pictures were made for a select circle of art lovers, they are difficult to decode. They are often complex and detailed, but we have no information about the images and little information about the first owner or about the setting where the paintings originally hung. In this sense, their socio-genesis interferes with an interpretation of their meanings.

I studied the *kraamkamers* in an effort to understand changes in the selection of subject and ways of seeing. Which events did painters think worthwhile to depict, and what kind of pictures did buyers want as decoration for their walls? Were there any changes in the events depicted and sold? We were especially interested in the social aspects of *kraamkamer* paintings, rather than attending to symbolic meanings, although some of them do have hidden significations.

In studying pictures of about fifty *kraamkamers*, the most important issue was the degree of privacy illustrated, as well as changes over time, especially those showing the relationships between families and the community. The degree of privacy was deduced from the presence, number, and activity of neighbors, relatives, servants, and dry nurses. Moreover, we examined the confined or open nature of the scenes by looking at the presence of windows and doors; were they open or closed, and did they give a view on the world outside? A comparison between the earlier and the later pictures yields some remarkable shifts in those respects.

The pictures of the earlier seventeenth century depict community visits of neighbors, relatives, and acquaintances. At first, the scenes are crowded with people, but over the century, the number decreases. Of the fifty *kraamkamer* paintings, there is a maximum of nineteen adults portrayed, but the average number is seven adults. For the later *kraamkamers* by Jan Horemans (1682–1759), the maximum number of adults is ten, and the average is seven. Some pictures only depict women, who are busy with the baby and the mother in bed. When the mother is shown mixing with the visitors, she is lost in the crowd of other women who are helping her. They are drying clothes in front of the fire, preparing food for the mother, and washing and feeding the baby. Other pictures depict some women sitting together and talking while showing the baby to each other. This gathering is reminiscent of the gossip scene in the above-mentioned play of *Zaartje Jans*. When men are present, they are drinking and eating, sometimes together with their wives. In some pictures, people are entering or leaving the house; others provide a view of the world outside the room or even outside the house.

The *kraamkamers* of Cornelis Troost, painted between 1737 and 1746, are different in two respects: they are more intimate as well as less crowded. Troost did not represent the social festivities, but rather the intimate circle around mother and infant after the birth. The setting was a well-to-do nuclear family, often of wealth and festivity. The intimacy of the subject continues the trend towards a decreasing number of depicted figures. Apart from one picture showing nine people, all of Troost's *kraamkamers* contain five or fewer people. The average number of adults is four. In all of his pictures, the mother, baby, and dry nurse, the reviled precursor of maternity care, are present; in some of them, the father, the doctor, a servant, or a girl may also be depicted. The mother is always lying in bed, sometimes with the father sitting near her and sometimes with the doctor, who is usually portrayed farcically. The dry nurse is feeding the baby, and sometimes the father or a young girl is looking over her shoulder. In some pictures a servant is bringing

in or preparing food. Help is given by persons who seem to be employees of
the parents. Troost's pictures are closed in the sense that he does not let us
catch a glimpse of the world outside. If the door is open, we see nothing more
than the suggestion of a garden; if there are any windows, they do not dis-
close a clear view. A comparison among earlier pictures and the pictures of
Troost seems to point to a shift in choice of subject and in representation
of the scene. It is not clear whether this shift was characteristic of Troost or
of the period, but the nuclear family scene and Troost's way of representing it
say something about changing preferences in certain elite circles.

The seventeenth-century Dutch attached much value to birth and childbed,
and were interested in representations of these scenes. Painters portrayed
such events at first as social gatherings, with an important communal function. Later on, they showed childbed scenes as private happenings, enacted
within the nuclear family circle. This change may indicate a change in artistic
style, or it may mirror a change of interest for painters and purchasers and a
different context of production. It is possible that the earlier pictures were
made for an anonymous market, for a simple and sober public, while the intimate *kraamkamers* of Troost were meant for a select and sophisticated
circle.

If the decrease in the number of depicted persons and changed relationships among participants—from help by many neighbors to help by one or
more paid assistants, such as dry nurse and maid—are indications of the
privatization of the nuclear family, one may conclude from the pictures of
kraamkamers that in Dutch towns this process was occurring during the seventeenth and the first half of the eighteenth centuries. If the small nuclear
families represented by Troost are indicative of the standards of the urban
elite around him, this process of privatization had in the 1730s and 1740s
been advanced to such a degree that the socio-genesis of the *modern* intimate
family in these circles had become a fact.

CONCLUSION

The varied materials we have used to study the development of Dutch birth
and childbed arrangements may not provide incontrovertible evidence when
examined individually, but taken together, they reinforce each other to provide an informed image of early childbed customs. In the Netherlands, the
nuclear family became separated from the wider community during the seventeenth and first half of the eighteenth centuries. In the urban elites, where
the making of the modern family had started, the process had been more or
less completed around 1740.

One aspect of the nuclearization of family life was the privatization of childbirth and childbed, which became increasingly intimate events, including only
parents, siblings, and helpers. Births came to lose much of their former communal character. The *kraamhuis* became less accessible for relatives and

neighbors, protecting mother and child, and secluding them from the wider community. The increased importance of a birth and its privatization are reflected in pictures of childbed scenes. Such events were deemed worthy subjects and viewed as decorative portrayals of the nuclear family. As such, they probably functioned as models for family life.

In the work of Edward Shorter (1975) and Lawrence Stone (1979, 1977), England comes to the fore as the country where the modern family first arose. According to Stone, whose research applies to the rich families of merchants and *professionals* in the towns, the modern family came into being in England at the end of the seventeenth century. From our research into the Netherlands, we conclude that the Dutch urban elite families nuclearized in the last decennia of the seventeenth and the first decennia of the eighteenth centuries. For this reason, a comparison of the modernization of family life and birth arrangements between England and the Netherlands would be worthwhile.[40] In any event, the nuclearization and privatization of the Dutch family seem to have taken place earlier than in France and central Europe.

Along with the early nuclearization of the family, a domestic emphasis is characteristic for seventeenth- and eighteenth-century Dutch family life. Within this context, childbirth became an important and privatized event. In the twentieth century, traditional domestic arrangements for *normal* birth and childbed were maintained, along with modern, medicalized arrangements in case of *pathology*. This dual obstetric system is in harmony with Dutch domestic family culture, which has a long tradition, as well as with the modern character of contemporary Dutch society.

NOTES

1. The remaining mothers not only give birth in the hospital, but spend their childbed there as well.

2. The Dutch concept of *gezelligheid* is deeply embedded in the culture and is difficult to translate. It corresponds to a mixture of warmth, security, and acceptance, and is an essential characteristic of Dutch family life.

3. The German sociologist Ferdinand Tönnies (1887) described the social changes caused by industrialization, commercialization, and urbanization as a transition from the traditional, rural community, the *Gemeinschaft*, to a differentiated society, the *Gesellschaft*.

4. Anderson, Michael, *Approaches to the History of the Western Family, 1500–1914* (London: Macmillan, 1980): 40–48.

5. For example, Pollock, Linda, *Forgotten Children: Parent-Child Relations from 1500–1900* (Cambridge: Cambridge University Press, 1983); Wrightson, Keith, *English Society, 1580–1680* (New Brunswick, N.J.: Rutgers University Press, 1982).

6. This chapter deals with the *Republiek der Zeven Verenigde Provinciën* from the end of the sixteenth century to the end of the eighteenth century. The *Republiek* comprised a smaller and less varied territory than the Netherlands today. Nevertheless, the *Republiek*, with Holland as its core, may be seen as the predecessor of the

present Dutch nation-state. For that reason, I use *the Netherlands* as synonymous with the *Republiek*.

7. Shorter, Edward, *The Making of the Modern Family* (London: Collins, 1975).

8. Schama, Simon, *The Embarrassment of Riches; An Interpretation of Dutch Culture in the Golden Age* (New York: Knopf, 1987).

9. Haks, Donald, *Huwelijk en gezin in Holland in de 17de en 18de eeuw* (Utrecht: Hes, 1985).

10. Burke, Peter, *Venice and Amsterdam* (London: Temple Smith, 1974): 87–88. *See* also Olsen, Donald J., "Urbanity, modernity, and liberty," *Two Essays on Urban History and Amsterdam* (Amsterdam: Center for Metropolitan Research, 1988/1990): 30–34.

11. Goudsblom, Johan, *Dutch Society* (New York: Random House, 1967).

12. Goudsblom, Johan, *Taal en sociale werkelijkheid. Sociologische stukken* (Amsterdam: Meulenhoff, 1988).

13. A family consisting of married partners and their children, without any or with little contacts with relatives, in which individual interest predominated and patriarchal authority was no longer accepted. Haks, Donald, *Huwelijk en gezin in Holland in de 17e en 18de eeuw* (Utrecht: Hes, 1985): 1.

14. Comparing the recruitment of the elite in Amsterdam and Venice, Peter Burke sees a relation between the patterns of social stratification and the kind of education current in those societies. Amsterdam seems to have been a more open, achievement-oriented society, particularly in the early days of the *Republiek*, with individual, geographical and social mobility, both upwards and downwards (Burke, note 7 above, pp. 16–33, 94–100). This achievement orientation probably had implications for the way parents raised their offspring and, more generally, for their attitude towards children. Under such conditions, the social chances of children were affected by their parents, and investments by parents counted heavily in the future of young adults. Maintaining good relations with offspring was a way of protecting the family capital or the family business. Goudsblom (note 12, p. 37) states that money and solidity were in this period of greater importance than titles and pedigrees. Ella Snoep-Reitsma ("Verschuivende betekenissen van zeventiende eeuwse Nederlandse genre-voostellingen" [Utrecht, 1975], thesis) also sees a connection between the special interest of seventeenth-century Dutch parents in their children and the capitalist or protocapitalist Dutch society of that period.

15. Women in labor and childbed were not rigorously banished to special places, as was the case with the Arapesh of New Guinea, where birth took place outside the village, in the "bad place" also reserved for excretion, menstrual huts, and foraging pigs. Mead, Margaret, *Sex and Temperament in Three Primitive Societies* (New York: William Morrow, 1935).

16. According to the Hebrew-Christian tradition, births were seen as unclean and shame-ridden because of sexual implications. Mead, Margaret, and Niles Newton, "Cultural patterning of perinatal behavior," in *Childbearing: Its Social and Psychological Aspects*, Richardson, A., and Alan R. Guttmacher (eds.) (Williams and Wilkins, 1967): 169–177.

17. Quoted in van Lieburg, M. J., "Het verloskundig onderwijs aan de klinische school (1828–1867)," in *Rijkskweekschool voor vroedvrouwen te Rotterdam 1882–*

1982, Scholte, E., et al. (eds.) (Leidschendam: Ministerie van Volksgezondheid en Milieuhygiene, 1982): 22.

18. Shorter, Edward, *A History of Women's Bodies* (New York: Basic Books, 1982): 53–54.

19. Jacobs, Aletta, *Herinneringen* (Nijmegen: SUN, 1978, originally published in 1924): 51–52.

20. Until recently, there has been a distinction between the more traditional countryside and the cities. In the countryside, births take place at home more often than in the cities. Among women living in villages with fewer than 5,000 inhabitants in the Netherlands in 1962, 79 percent had their babies at home and, in 1979, 46.9 percent. Of women living in cities of more than 500,000 inhabitants in 1962, 47 percent had their babies at home and, in 1979, 12 percent. van Daalen, Rineke, "De groei van de ziekenhuisbevalling: Nederland en het buitenland," *Amsterdams Sociologisch Tijdschrift* 15:3 (December 1988): 431.

21. van der Woude, A. M., "De omvang en samenstelling van de huishouding in Nederland in het verleden," in *Economische ontwikkeling en sociale emancipatie*, Geurts, P.A.M., and F.A.M. Messing (eds.) (Den Haag: Nijhoff, 1977): 211, 212.

22. van Idsinga, J. H. *Staatsrecht der Vereenigde Nederlanden* (Leeuwarden: Ferwerda, 1758): 325–330. It would be worthwhile to compare the development of those regulations in different towns and countries.

23. See J. Le Francq van Berkhey, *Natuurlijke Historie van Holland III* (Amsterdam: Yntema & Tieboel, 1773): 1248–1250.

24. Lunsingh Scheurleer, Th. H., "Enkele oude Nederlandse kraamgbruiken," *Antiek*, 6 (1971/1972): 314.

25. Huizinga, Johan, *Herfsttij der Middeleeuwen* (Groningen: Wolters-Noordhoff, 1984, originally published in 1919): 48.

26. Kelderman, Cornelis, *Ampt Ende Plicht Der Vroed-Vrouwen* (Alphen aan den Rijn/Brussel: Stafleu, 1981, originally published in 1697): 2, 3.

27. Schrader, C. G., *Memory Boeck van de Vrouwens. het Notitieboek van een Friese vroedvrouw 1693–1745* (Amsterdam: Rodopi, 1984): 202.

28. Asschelijn, Tomas, *Kraam-bed of kandeel-maal van Zaartje Jans* (Amsterdam: Alexander Lintman, 1684). Many different versions of this play have been put into circulation, some not authorized by the author.

29. With respect to bylaws, *see* Schotel, G.D.F., *Het Oud-Hollandsch huisgezin der zeventiende eeuw* (Haarlem: Kruseman, 1867). *See* also Spierenburg, Pieter, *De verbroken betovering: Mentaliteitsgeschie denis van preindustrieel Europa* (Hilversum: Verloren, 1990): 312–314; Le Francq van Berkhey, J., *Natuurlijke Historie van Holland III* (Amsterdam: Yntema & Tieboel, 1773): 1248–1250.

30. The following list is not exhaustive, but gives an idea of the number of Dutch painters who depicted one or more *kraamkamers*: Anthonie Palamedesz (1601–1673); Adriaen van Ostade (1610–84); Gerard Dou (1613–75); Quiringh G. Brekelenkam (ca. 1620–68); Hieronymus Janssens (1624–93); Cornelis de Man (1624–84); Jan H. Steen (1626–79); Pieter de Hoogh (1624–84); Gabriel Metsu (1629–67); C. Bisschop (1630–74); Cornelis P. Bega (ca. 1632–64); Matthijs Naiveu (1647–1721); Jan Luyken (1649–1712); Richard Brakenburgh (1650–1702); Jan J. Horemans (1682–1759); Cornelis Troost (1696–1750).

31. Provisional research confirms the suggestion that Dutch painters had a special

interest in *kraamkamers*. *See* Mullerheim, Robert, *Die Wochenstube in der Kunst* (Stuttgart: Ferdinand Enke, 1904). Mainly Dutch and Italian *kraam* scenes have been reproduced.

32. In his quantification of the production of paintings in Holland during the *Republiek*, A. M. van der Woude states that the total production comprised between 5 and 10 million pieces. He assesses the total number of paintings in collections in Holland between 1580 and 1800 at about 18 million. "De schilderijproduktie in Holland tijdens de Republiek. Een poging tot kwantificatie," in Dagevos, J. C. et al., *Kunstzaken: Particulier initiatief en overheidsbeleid in de wereld van de beeldende kunst* (Kampen: Kok Agora, 1991): 30–35.

33. Van Deursen, A. Th., *Mensen van klein vermogen: Het "Kopergeld" van de Gouden Eeuw* (Amsterdam: Bert Bakker, 1991, originally published in 1978). Van der Woude, note 32 above, pp. 45–46.

34. Haak, B., *Hollandse schilders in de Gouden Eeuw* (Amsterdam: Meulenhoff/ Landshoff, 1984): 85–98.

35. Haverkamp Begemann, quoted in Haak, ibid., p. 71.

36. Goudsblom, Johan, "Problemen bij de sociologische studie van romans," in *Romantropologie*, van Bremen, Jan, et al. (eds.) (Amsterdam: Antropologisch-Sociologisch Centrum, 1979): 8.

37. van Deursen, *see* note 21 above, p. 89. The traditional vision is that the court did not contribute significant amounts of patronage, but recently the role of the court of the *stadhouder* has been brought to the fore. *See* Kempers, Bram, "Opdrachtgevers, verzamelaars en kopers. Visies op kunst in Holland tijdens de Republiek," *Holland* 23, 4/5 (1991): 197, 201. In interpreting the *kraakamer* paintings, Kempers' article has often been used.

38. From van Gool's description of Troost's life and career, it seems that most of his art was done on contract, sometimes commissioned by a public institution like the Godtshuizen or the Collegium Medicum, and sometimes by art lovers. van Gool, J., *De nieuwe schouburg der Nederlantsche kunstschilders en schilderessen II* ('s-Gravenhage, 1751): 243–252.

39. For example, C. Ploos van Amstel, P. L. de Neufville. Niemeijer, J. W., *Cornelis Troost 1696–1750* (Assen: Van Gorcum, 1973): 320, 323.

40. Le Francq van Berkhey (*see* note 23 above) commented that England was a modern country because it was the first one where the old-fashioned practice of swaddling was abolished (1773).

II

THE OBSTETRIC SYSTEM AND THE QUALITY OF CARE

5

Selection as the Basis of Obstetric Care in the Netherlands

Pieter E. Treffers

INTRODUCTION

A Dutch obstetrician traveling abroad finds himself questioned repeatedly about the remarkable phenomenon of home births in the Netherlands. Moreover, many people seek information about Dutch obstetric care by writing letters or visiting the country. Indeed, contrary to other European countries and to all developed countries in the Western world, the Netherlands still preserves a system of obstetric care that includes a considerable number of home deliveries. Home births seem to be the most distinctive feature of Dutch obstetrics, and the system of care has often been admired or condemned because of this single feature. Home deliveries constitute only a conspicuous detail of the system of care, however; more basic is the selection of pregnant women into risk groups and early identification of obstetric pathology. It is only on the basis of selection that the system of care prevailing in the Netherlands can be properly understood and assessed.

LEVELS OF CARE

As in other fields of medicine, obstetric care in the Netherlands can be divided into three levels. Primary care comprises the care given by midwife and general practitioner. Midwives are fully qualified and licensed to provide independent care during normal pregnancy and childbirth. At the beginning of pregnancy, the woman usually visits her general practitioner. He refers her for prenatal and natal care to a midwife and, sometimes, in cases of apparent

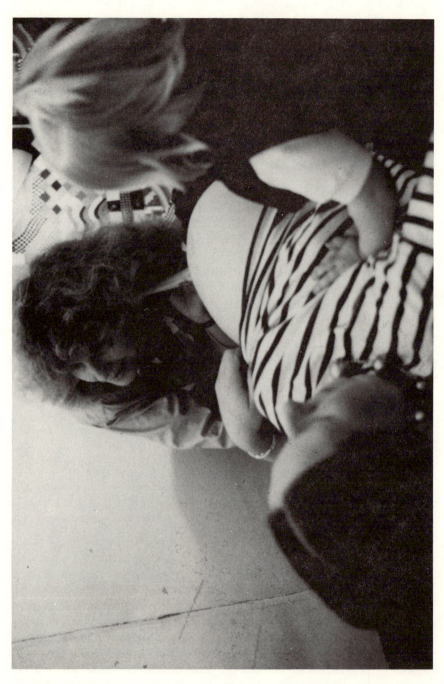

Midwife Astrid Limburg listening to fetal heart sounds with "trumpet." Used by permission of Astrid Limburg.

obstetrical or medical pathology, to an obstetrician. Sometimes the woman goes directly to the midwife. In regions where there are no midwives (the less densely populated and more remote parts of the country), primary obstetric care is given by the general practitioner.

Secondary prenatal and natal care is provided by an obstetrician who accepts referrals from a midwife or general practitioner, either during pregnancy or during labor. Referrals are made because of increased risk for the mother or the fetus, or because there is some sign of medical or obstetrical pathology. The obstetrician may already have treated some women for infertility or other gynecological disorders. In such cases, he may decide to refer these women to the midwife when they are pregnant, or to keep them under his own care because he considers them at higher risk of complications.

Tertiary care is given in perinatal centers, predominantly in the eight university hospitals. Obstetric care is given in close cooperation with neonatologists in a neonatal intensive care unit, with other subspecialists of pediatrics and internal medicine, and with clinical geneticists. The main indications for referral to a tertiary center are threatening preterm labor before thirty-two weeks of pregnancy, severe pre-eclampsia or eclampsia, severe fetal growth retardation, or suspicion of congenital malformations of the fetus.

Anyone with an income under a certain level (about 65 percent of the total population) falls within the group compulsorily insured by National Health Service, which includes all medical and obstetrical risks. The insurance contribution is deducted from individuals' salaries. The 35 percent of the population with the highest incomes are expected to insure themselves privately, and almost all of them are insured. The National Health Service and some of the private insurance companies remunerate specialist care only after referral by a general practitioner or midwife, and then only in cases of medical or obstetric pathology. Obstetric primary care by a general practitioner is remunerated by the compulsory insurance only if there are no midwives in the neighborhood. This means that almost every citizen is insured for medical and obstetric care, but only at the level considered appropriate.

SELECTION PROCEDURE

The different types of care available for different persons result in a selection procedure to decide who is in need of secondary or tertiary care. The Dutch system strongly favors primary care; prenatal care and care during childbirth by obstetricians will be remunerated only if there are medical or obstetrical reasons for it. Those who decide whether childbirth is likely to be safely conducted by primary-care attendants, either at home or in the hospital, are the midwife and the general practitioner. They need guidelines to distinguish who is in need of specialist care. As early as the 1960s, Gerrit-Jan Kloosterman devised a list of medical indications for specialist care that he included in the 1973 Dutch textbook on obstetrics and gynecology he edited.

The list, translated into English by M.J.N.C. Keirse (1982), is not comprehensive. It provided guidelines for which pregnant women should be delivered by obstetricians in a hospital and which types of obstetric pathology warrant remuneration by health insurance for specialist care. But supervising compliance with the regulations laid down in the medical indications list was not strictly enforced. In practice, various reasons for specialist care were honored at the discretion of the medical advisor of a particular health insurance.

In the early 1980s, some dissatisfaction arose about the implementation of the list of medical indications, especially among primary-care health workers (midwives and general practitioners) and among health-care providers. The percentage of medical indications for specialist care had increased considerably (from 26 percent in 1971 to 46 percent in 1979), with a large variation among regions (from 40 percent to 80 percent). This resulted in the establishment of a commission whose task was to advise on the revision of the list of medical indications by the Medical Insurance Board (*Ziekenfondsraad*). In 1987, the committee published its final report, which recommended a selection process based on four criteria, in case of an increased risk that would possibly necessitate specialist or hospital care:

1. The increased risk of complications and their nature and gravity
2. The possibilities of primary and secondary care to prevent these complications
3. The possibilities of primary and secondary care to detect complications in time
4. The possibilities of primary and secondary care to intervene adequately in case these complications occur.

The committee classifies pregnant women with one or more of a large number of risk factors to one of the following groups, based on these criteria:

A. The woman will receive primary care; the confinement may take place at home or in the hospital.
B. The woman will be referred to the obstetrician for consultation. After his or her advice, the midwife or general practitioner will decide on subsequent care. The consultation may lead to a decision for hospital delivery under the care of midwife or general practitioner.
C. The woman will be referred to the obstetrician for secondary care; confinement takes place in the hospital.

The various risk factors and the assignment to one of the groups A, B, or C are listed in the Appendix.

The report of the commission on the revision of the list of medical indications was intended to put a stop to the increasing number of medical indications for specialist care. It met strong opposition from the Board of Obstetricians and Gynecologists. Although the report was accepted by the Medical Insurance Board (*Ziekenfondsraad*) and by the organizations of midwives and general practitioners, the large majority of obstetricians opposed the report and refused to comply with the conclusions. The strongest opposition centered on the ultimate decision for recommending care being in the hands of midwife or general practitioner in doubtful cases, after the obstetrician's consultation (group B), and the possibility that in cases of medium risk, the midwife or general practitioner may conduct a delivery on medical indication in the hospital.

Currently, there is no generally approved list of medical indications, and practitioners of various disciplines interpret the concept of "medical indications" in a slightly different way. Although not often admitted openly, the discussion about medical indications is often influenced by the income of the various participants.

Although on a national level there is no agreement about the system of medical indications, in practice, in the various regions cooperation among the different obstetric practitioners involved (midwives, general practitioners, and obstetricians) is usually good.

CARE DURING LABOR AND DELIVERY

The latest data for the type of professional care selected for labor and delivery are from 1989. In that year, midwives attended childbirth in 45.7 percent of the cases, obstetricians in 43 percent, and general practitioners in 11.3 percent. These percentages indicate the care chosen at the time of birth. The women attended by obstetricians include those referred during pregnancy as well as those referred during the second stage of labor (instrumental deliveries: forcipal or vacuum extractions). Between 10 and 20 percent of the pregnant women under the care of midwives are referred to the obstetrician during pregnancy, and an equal percentage during labor. Approximately 80 percent of pregnant women start their pregnancies under the care of midwives or general practitioners.

In the same year, 1989, 33.4 percent of all children were born at home (*Centraal Bureau voor de Statistiek*, 1992). This figure was 35.8 percent in 1978 (after a steady decline following the war), and then stabilized at the level of 35 percent, with a slight decrease since 1987. These figures indicate that at the beginning of labor, nearly 70 percent of all women still receive primary care by midwives or general practitioners; more than half of these women are then at home.

During labor and delivery, maternal and fetal surveillance by the midwife and general practitioner is different from surveillance by the obstetrician. In high-risk cases, surveillance by the obstetrician is usually by electronic monitoring; in many hospitals this is supplemented by fetal blood sampling, if necessary. The woman in labor is usually in bed. Surveillance by the midwife in low-risk cases is more liberal: Fetal monitoring is by intermittent auscultation with a monauricular stethoscope or a Doppler apparatus, the woman is free to move around during labor, and if she is at home, she may take a shower or a bath. Delivery may take place in the upright or horizontal position, according to her wishes.

The selection procedure, aimed at identifying risks and signs of pathology during pregnancy, is continued during labor and delivery. Symptoms such as meconium-stained amniotic fluid, abnormalities of the fetal heart rate, or profuse bleeding are indications for referral to the obstetrician. If the woman is still at home, the decision to refer her to the obstetrician will be made somewhat earlier than in the hospital, because transportation of a woman in labor to a nearby hospital takes about half an hour. On the other hand, the decision to consult an obstetrician if the first or the second stage of labor is progressing slowly is made more often when the woman is already in the hospital. All in all, referrals are somewhat more frequent if the woman starts labor in the hospital than when she starts at home.

CARE DURING THE FIRST WEEK POSTPARTUM

In home confinement, a maternity home-care assistant usually assists the midwife or general practitioner during childbirth. Thereafter, the maternity home-care assistant takes care of mother and child daily, advises the mother and the father on the care of the newborn, breastfeeding, and plays an important role in checking the health of mother and child. The midwife and general practitioner supervise her, and may refer mother or child to the obstetrician or the pediatrician in case of pathology. Of the infants born at home, between 3 and 4 percent are referred to the pediatrician during the first week of life; referrals of the mother are rare, less than 1 percent.

In hospital confinement, mother and child usually go home within six to twelve hours, if their condition is satisfactory. They receive the same care at home as is offered after home births. If there are any complications, they stay in the hospital as long as necessary. Hospital care during the first week postpartum is remunerated by insurance providers only if there was a medical indication for such (*see* Appendix).

EFFECTIVENESS OF THE SELECTION PROCEDURE

There are some difficulties in evaluating the effectiveness of the system of care in the Netherlands. Nationwide detailed statistical data about the results of obstetric care are lacking, although some general statistical data are available from the Central Bureau of Statistics (number of births, liveborns and stillborns, place of birth, etc.). Moreover, there are two separate obstetric data bases: The first contains data about secondary care by obstetricians in the hospital; the second comprises care by midwives, at home and in the hospital. General practitioners do not collect data about obstetric care. Up to now, it has not been possible to link the two data bases together, and the outcomes of pregnancies of women referred by the midwife to the obstetrician are available only in the data base of secondary care. The data bases do not allow full evaluation of the outcome of primary care nationwide. Apparently one of the characteristics of the system of care, the small scale of the independent practices of midwives, general practitioners, and obstetricians providing medical and obstetrical care in the countryside, hampers the collection of nationwide reliable statistical information. This drawback compels us to base our evaluation of the system of care on research projects carried out on samples of the population.

The most extensive research thus far has been the Wormerveer study (van Alten, Eskes, and Treffers, 1989; M. Eskes, 1989). This long-term prospective investigation focused on the effectiveness of care in an independent midwives' practice in a small suburban region north of Amsterdam. The study comprised 7,980 women consecutively booked at the midwives' practice over fourteen years (1969–1983), with a complete follow-up of their pregnancies, deliveries, and the 8,055 infants they gave birth to. One of the aims of the study was to evaluate the selection procedure by the midwives. Of four well-defined risk groups (twins, preterm deliveries less than thirty-seven weeks, growth-retarded infants $\leq 2.3^{\text{rd}}$ percentile, and breech deliveries), the data showed how many were referred in time and therefore delivered under the care of the obstetrician, and how many of the infants were born under the exclusive care of a midwife. Of the twins, 91 percent were referred in time, and 9 percent were delivered by a midwife. Preterm infants were referred in 80 percent of the cases, and 20 percent were delivered under the care of a midwife. The large majority of these (17 percent) were infants born after more than thirty-six weeks during the first part of the study, when referral because of preterm labor at a gestational age of thirty-six weeks was not yet common practice. The detection and referral of growth-retarded infants was not very effective: 59 percent were referred before birth, and 41 percent were born under the exclusive care of a midwife. Of the women having a child in breech presentation, 94 percent were referred in time, and 6 percent were delivered by the midwife. The deliveries in breech presentation by the midwives were uneventful; there were no deaths, and at the age of five years, the children were healthy.

Although the selection procedure was not perfect, in three of the four risk groups, the large majority of women were referred in time, so that the delivery could take place in a hospital by the obstetrician. During the fourteen-year period of the study, the selection of twins, threatening preterm labor, and breech presentation improved considerably. It is expected that since the study was done, improvements in detecting twins and breech presentations will have been made because of the advancement in ultrasound technology that is also available to midwives. Although early diagnosis of fetal growth retardation remains a problem, this diagnosis is difficult for obstetricians, too.

M. P. Springer (1991) performed a comparable study on the effectiveness of obstetric care of thirteen general practitioners in 1980–84. The retrospective study could not locate about 10 percent of the pregnant women. With respect to the selection procedure of the 1,841 women in this study, the conclusion was that in the four risk groups (twins, preterm birth, fetal growth retardation, and breech presentation), the accuracy of prenatal screening by the general practitioner was comparable to the results of the midwives in the Wormerveer study.

EFFECTIVENESS OF THE CARE

In the early 1980s, two Dutch studies were published comparing umbilical cord pH values and standardized neurological examination among infants born at home and in the hospital under the care of midwives and obstetricians (T.K.A.B. Eskes, Jongsma, and Houx, 1981; Lievaart and De Jong, 1982). The umbilical cord pH is a measure of hypoxia during birth, a low pH corresponding with more severe hypoxia, and the neurological examination gives an assessment of the condition of the central nervous system of the newborn infant. The groups studied were small. The first study looked at 170 infants, eighty-five born at home and eighty-five in the hospital, and the second study included eighty-five deliveries attended by midwives and twenty-seven conducted by obstetricians. Both studies concluded that the results in those infants born under specialist care appeared to be significantly better than in those under midwives' care. These studies have been discussed widely and criticized on methodological grounds (Monagle, 1983; Treffers, van Alten, and Pel, 1983). The reliability of cord pH values depends largely on strict standardization of cord clamping, sampling time, and blood storage (Pel and Treffers, 1983). Late clamping, delay in sampling, and longer storage of blood samples all cause a decrease in pH values, erroneously suggesting severe hypoxia during birth. The necessary standardization was not guaranteed during routine obstetric care in these studies, especially not in the home deliveries. Moreover, in the first study, instrumental deliveries were excluded from the category of hospital deliveries, despite the authors' conclusion that the results of home deliveries could have been improved by instrumental interventions. In the second study, eighty-five deliveries attended by midwives were compared with only twenty-seven deliveries by obstetricians. The twenty-seven deliveries originated from a group of forty-five women, and only cursory data about the eighteen excluded women were provided.

In the Wormerveer study (van Alten, Eskes, and Treffers, 1989; M. Eskes, 1989), perinatal mortality was examined, including all stillbirths and neonatal deaths within one week of birth for infants with a birth weight ≥ 500 g.), and infant morbidity was measured by admission rate to the hospital and by the number of convulsions in the first week of life. All infants were followed up for at least four weeks, and infant mortality was registered up to one year of age. In a subgroup of the total population of newborns (175 consecutive bookings in 1982), the umbilical artery pH was recorded, and a neurological examination (Prechtl and Beintema, 1964) was performed using strictly standardized methods.

Of the eighty-nine total perinatal deaths, fifteen occurred in the group of 6,625 infants born to mothers selected as low-risk cases during pregnancy, all of whom started labor under the care of the midwife. Perinatal mortality in this group was 2.3 per 1,000. The remaining seventy-four perinatal deaths occurred in the group of 1,430 infants born to mothers selected as high-risk cases and referred to the obstetrician during pregnancy. Perinatal mortality in this group was 51.7 per 1,000; in the total group of 8,055 infants, perinatal mortality amounted to 11.1 per 1,000.

Convulsions in the first week of life occurred in twelve of the 8,055 children (1.5 per 1,000); in seven cases, the convulsions occurred in term infants during the first forty-eight hours after birth (0.9 per 1,000). J. Dennis and I. Chalmers (1982), who proposed this incidence of convulsions as a standard for measuring the quality of perinatal care, found in Great Britain an incidence of 4.2 convulsions per 1,000 births and 1.7 per 1,000 births in term infants within forty-eight hours of life. In an Irish study, the incidence of convulsions was 3.0 per 1,000 births (MacDonald et al., 1985).

Special attention was paid to strict standardization of umbilical cord pH determination and neurological examination of the newborn infants. All infants born from mothers seen at the midwives' practice in a fixed period of time in 1982 were included in the investigation. A member of the team of investigators was present at all deliveries; his or her only duty was the clamping of the cord, sampling of blood immediately after birth, and determination of the pH as soon as possible. This research therefore was independent of routine obstetric care by the midwife.

The results were remarkable. Contrary to the investigations mentioned before, the pH values of the infants born under the exclusive care of a midwife were very good. Those obtained from first-born infants were higher than the values found by others (T.K.A.B. Eskes, Jongsma, and Houx, 1981; Sykes et al., 1982) in hospital deliveries attended by obstetricians. Higher pH values correspond with better oxygen supply during labor and delivery. The pH values and the neurological condition of first-born infants born under the care of midwives were significantly better than the pH values and the neurological condition of first-born infants born under the care of the obstetrician after referral of the mother during pregnancy (Knuist, Eskes, and van Alten, 1987; M. Eskes, Knuist, and van Alten, 1987). Presumably these differences are not caused by bad obstetric care by the obstetrician, but by the effectiveness of the selection procedure by the midwife leading to the referral of high-risk cases. The same holds true for the differences in perinatal mortality among the group of infants born under the care of a midwife and the group born under the care of the obstetrician.

In the Wormerveer study, the rate of intervention was extremely low. In the total group of 7,980 women, 110 (1.4 percent) had a Caesarean section. In the group selected as low-risk cases during pregnancy (6,613 women), there were only twenty-nine Caesarean sections (0.4 percent).

G. Berghs and E. Spanjaards (1988), in a study in the Nijmegen area, investigated 1,034 infants born to women classified as low-risk by neurological examination in the neonatal period. Some of the women were attended during pregnancy and delivery by a midwife (62 percent) or general practitioner (12 percent). The majority of these women delivered at home. About 26 percent of the women were attended by an obstetrician in a hospital. The neurological condition of the newborns did not differ in the cohorts attended by the midwives, general practitioners, and obstetricians. The main difference between the deliveries attended by obstetricians and those attended by midwives and general practitioners was a significantly higher rate of intervention by the obstetricians. The specialists used oxytocin for the induction or the acceleration of labor in 21.3 percent of the cases, compared with 14.8 percent in the general practitioner group and 4.5 percent in the midwife group. They performed episiotomies in 60.8 percent of the cases, compared with 54.8 percent in the general practitioner group and 35.1 percent in the midwife group, and they performed instrumental and operative deliveries in 16.0 percent of the cases, compared with 8.6 percent in the general practitioner group and 5.9 percent in the midwife group. The comparatively high number of interventions by obstetricians attending low-risk women during labor has been confirmed by Davis et al. in the United States (1991).

In a study of the obstetric care by general practitioners (Springer, 1991), which measured the quality of care according to perinatal mortality, timely referral to the obstetrician, and injury to the health of mother or child, the conclusion was that general practitioners provided good care.

MISUNDERSTANDING OF THE SELECTION PROCEDURE

People interested in the system of care from outside the Netherlands often find it difficult to appreciate the influence of selection on the outcome of pregnancies in subgroups of the population. For instance, visitors from other countries are sometimes amazed that perinatal mortality in our university department in Amsterdam is among the highest in the Netherlands. In a seven-year period, 1983–89, perinatal mortality in our department (≥500 g. and ≥24 weeks' gestational duration, stillborns and neonatal deaths up to four weeks after birth) was forty-five per 1,000 (Wolf, 1991). This very high mortality is not caused by bad perinatal care, but by a high concentration of pathology in a regional perinatal center. For instance, in 1983–89, the incidence of preterm birth (less than thirty-seven weeks) in our department was 22 percent, whereas for very early preterm birth (less than thirty-two weeks) it was 10 percent. At the same time, perinatal mortality among infants whose births were attended by midwives at home and in hospitals was of the magnitude of 1–1.5 per 1,000. Perinatal mortality in our university department was therefore more than thirty times higher than mortality under primary care, because the women at extremely high risk were referred to the university hospital, whereas the women who delivered at home were selected as low-risk cases. The percentage of perinatal mortality in a general hospital providing secondary care is lower than in a university hospital, but higher than in home births.

A comparable misunderstanding is apparent in a recent report of the Royal College of Obstetricians and Gynaecologists in Great Britain (1992). The report comments on the system of obstetric care in the Netherlands and mentions the perinatal mortality figures of the Wormerveer study:

> The evidence from the Netherlands shows that if women are correctly categorised as low or high risk, the outcomes for both mother and child are favourable. However, if problems arise during pregnancy there is either insufficient flexibility or the interface between the two systems is inadequate to deal with them appropriately. The Wormerveer study reports a perinatal mortality in this group of 51.7 per 1000 which is clearly unacceptable.

Why is a high perinatal mortality unacceptable in a subgroup of the population if that subgroup has been selected precisely because of an anticipated high risk? The other subgroups of the same population show a very low mortality; the difference in mortality figures is evidence of a good selection system rather than of insufficient care.

In the Wormerveer study, women referred to the obstetrician because of (imminent) preterm labor were categorized as "referred during pregnancy" rather than "referred during labor." This was done to evaluate the effectiveness of the practice of midwives. Their main tasks are twofold: first to divide pregnant women into low- and high-risk groups, and second to attend normal deliveries after at least thirty-seven weeks of pregnancy. If labor starts earlier, their task is to recognize the signs of imminent labor and to refer the woman as a high-risk case to the hospital. If women who are hospitalized because labor started preterm were to be classified as "referred during labor," the mortality of this category would become very high, and this could be wrongly attributed to complications of labor attended by midwives at home. Signs of imminent preterm labor usually start unexpectedly during pregnancy and should therefore be classified as pathology of pregnancy. Only then is it possible to evaluate the care during labor at home by primary-care attendants without including all sorts of pathologies that occur during pregnancy. The classification into categories used in the Wormerveer study contributes to the high mortality figure in the group "referred during pregnancy," because perinatal mortality is by far the highest in preterm infants.

M. Tew and S.M.J. Damstra-Wijmenga (1991) also fail to understand the meaning of perinatal mortality figures. They state that perinatal mortality is caused by specialist care in hospitals, referring to the Dutch figures from the Wormerveer study. They consider the discrepancy between the perinatal mortality rate of 51.7 per 1,000 in the hospitalized group and 1.3 per 1,000 in the group remaining under the care of the midwives as "far too wide to be plausibly explained by the extra dangers of the complications." Their evaluation of the data is a misunderstanding of the impact of a selection procedure on mortality figures in subgroups of a population.

The German Society of Gynecology and Obstetrics published a report on home births (*Deutsche Gesellschaft für Gynäkologie und Geburtshilfe*, 1990) condemning home deliveries, partly based on the "Dutch experience," using a limited selection of the literature quoted out of context. The report states: "Observations in some cities in Germany show that perinatal mortality in home deliveries is as high as 20 per 1,000." In all of Germany, however, the figure is 0.7 per 1,000. The report does not provide any further information about the high mortality rate in home deliveries, and we suspect that the mortality figure does not represent the mortality in planned home deliveries, but contains complications occurring during pregnancy, including unexpected and unplanned home births. In a country where the number of planned home deliveries is very small, the outcome of unplanned home deliveries strongly influences the outcome of all home births. The German report therefore ignores the significance of the selection procedure in primary-care obstetrics.

DISCUSSION

From an epidemiological perspective, the selection of the population of pregnant women into high- and low-risk groups has considerable advantages if the diagnostic management during labor is also different in both groups. Diagnostic measures during labor and delivery are aimed primarily at the detection of fetal distress, and the most important diagnostic tool is the surveillance of fetal heart rate. The most sensitive method of fetal surveillance, electronic heart rate monitoring, can lead to unnecessary interventions, because the number of false-positive signs of fetal distress is relatively high, especially in a population with a low incidence of pathology. In such a population, a less sensitive method, intermittent auscultation, may be adequate to detect the rare cases of fetal distress in time. It has been shown that electronic fetal heart rate monitoring in low-risk cases may lead to unnecessary interventions (Prentice and Lind, 1987). In a high-risk population, however, with a much higher incidence of pathology, electronic monitoring may be useful for the early detection of fetal distress and may less often lead to unnecessary interventions. That the Caesarean section rate in the Netherlands is still relatively low (±7 percent nationwide) is probably related to the fact that the responsibility for the care of low-risk pregnant women (most women) is in the hands of midwives, professionals who do not routinely apply electronic monitoring, who are not qualified to intervene in the normal sequence of events, and who are dedicated to the preservation of physiology.

The outcomes of care in eighty-four birth centers in the United States, as reported by Rooks et al. in 1989, are to a large extent comparable with the results obtained in the Netherlands. In this study, the selection procedure for women at higher risk during prenatal care was similar—referrals during pregnancy were 18 percent, and referrals during labor and delivery were 15.8 percent of those admitted to birth centers. The rate of Caesarean section was low (4.4 percent).

One of the objects of investigation in the Wormerveer study was the presence of preventable factors in relation to the eighty-nine cases of perinatal mortality. An independent committee consisting of two obstetricians, a midwife, a general practitioner, a neonatologist, and a pathologist analyzed each case. The term "avoidable factors" stood for determinants that (in retrospect), if they had been avoided, might have prevented an adverse outcome. The committee concluded that in twenty-nine (33 percent) of the cases, avoidable factors were present to some extent. In seven cases, the skill of the midwife was at issue; the other twenty-two cases usually involved the management of the specialists (obstetricians and pediatricians). The intended place of delivery (home or hospital) played a minor and insignificant role in the discussion about avoidable factors (M. Eskes, 1989).

Although this chapter discussed the selection procedure carried out by primary-care attendants leading to categories of pregnant women at low and at high risk (possibly also a "medium-risk" category may be distinguished), another selection procedure is implemented by secondary-care workers (obstetricians): referral to tertiary perinatal centers. These centers, established during the last decades, accept referrals of patients at very high risk by obstetricians working in secondary care. Such referrals have gradually increased. The majority of infants with very short gestational ages and very low birth weights are now born in these perinatal centers. In a nationwide study of all live-born infants with a gestational age less than thirty-two weeks and/or a birth weight <1,500 g., it was shown that the neonatal mortality of infants born in level one or level two hospitals was significantly higher than of infants born in level 3 hospitals, the university perinatal centers (Verloove-Vanhorick et al., 1988). There are indications that the selection procedure for referral to tertiary centers has improved since 1983, but we do not have precise data.

Level 1 hospitals are the smaller regional hospitals; level 2 hospitals are larger training hospitals with more facilities for perinatal care.

It is possible that secondary care in the smaller level 1 hospitals, which have only a relatively small number of deliveries, is a weak point in the system of care. J. P. Mackenbach and P.L.M. Van Leengoed (1989), in an epidemiological study of regional perinatal mortality, found no correlation with regional hospitalization at delivery, but there was a negative correlation between regional perinatal mortality and the presence of a level 2 hospital in the neighborhood. Perinatal mortality was higher in communities having only a level 1 hospital. Possibly the small scale of some units of care in these hospitals is a handicap. More research is needed before we can draw any definite conclusions.

The Dutch system of obstetric care is divided into three levels. Primary care includes the option of home confinement. Essential in this division in levels of care is careful diagnosis in the prenatal, natal, and postnatal periods leading to the detection of risks and early signs of pathology, with consequent referral to a higher level of care. Because the incidence of pathologic phenomena in the categories selected accordingly is quite different, it is only logical that obstetric management is also diverse. This means that for the group of low-risk women, which is the majority, there is a large extent of freedom to experience the birth of their children in their own way, in the place of their own choice, with a minimum of medical interference and interventions (Treffers et al., 1990). It must be kept in mind, however, that this system is based not on freedom only, but on a meticulous selection system.

REFERENCES

Berghs, G., and E. Spanjaards. *De normale zwangerschap: Bevalling en Beleid.* Thesis, University of Nijmegen, 1988.

Centraal Bureau voor de Statistiek, *Births by obstetric assistance and place of delivery,* 1989. *Maandbericht Gezondheid* 1992: 13–28.

Davis, L. et al., *Cesarean section rates in low risk patients managed by nurse-midwives and obstetricians.* XIII World Congress of Gynaecology and Obstetrics (FIGO), abstract no. 0136. Singapore, 1991.

Dennis, J., and I. Chalmers, "Very early neonatal seizure rate: a possible epidemiological indicator of the quality of perinatal care," *British Journal of Obstetrics and Gynaecology,* vol. 89, (1982): 418–426.

Deutsche Gesellschaft für Gynäkologie und Geburtshilfe, *Stellungnahme der Deutschen Gesellschaft für Gynäkologie und Geburtshilfe zur Hausgeburtshilfe.* Amberg-Oberpfalz, 1990.

Eskes, M., M. Knuist, and D. van Alten, "Neurologisch onderzoek bij pasgeborenen in een verloskundigenpraktijk," *Nederlands Tijdschrift voor Geneeskunde,* vol. 131 (1987): 1040–1043.

Eskes, M., *Het Wormerveer onderzoek. Meerjarenonderzoek naar de kwaliteit van de verloskundige zorg rond een vroedvrouwenpraktijk.* Thesis, University of Amsterdam, 1989.

Eskes, T.K.A.B., H. W. Jongsma, and P.C.W. Houx, "Umbilical cord gases in home deliveries versus hospital-based deliveries," *Journal of Reproductive Medicine,* vol. 26 (1981): 405–408.

Keirse, M.J.N.C., "Interaction between primary and secondary antenatal care, with particular reference to the Netherlands," in Enkin, M., and I. Chalmers (eds.) *Effectiveness and Satisfaction in Antenatal Care.* (London: Spastics International Medical Publications, Heinemann Medical Books, 1982): 222–233.

Kloosterman, G. J., "Medische indicaties voor specialistische behandeling," in *De voortplanting van de mens. Leerboek voor obstetrie en gynaecologie.* Bussum: Centen, (1973): 732–735.

Knuist, M., M. Eskes, and D. van Alten, "De pH van het arteriële navelstrengbloed van pasgeborenen bij door vroedvrouwen geleide bevallingen," *Nederlands Tijdschrift voor Geneeskunde,* vol. 131 (1987): 362–365.

Lievaart, M., and P. A. De Jong, "Neonatal morbidity in deliveries conducted by midwives and gynecologists: a study of the system of obstetric care prevailing in The Netherlands," *American Journal of Obstetrics and Gynecology,* vol. 144 (1982): 376–386.

MacDonald, D. et al., "The Dublin randomized controlled trial of intrapartum fetal heart rate monitoring," *American Journal of Obstetrics and Gynecology,* vol. 152 (1985): 524–539.

Mackenbach, J. P., and P.L.M. Van Leengoed, "Regionale verschillen in perinatale sterfte: het verband met enkele aspecten van de zorg rond de geboorte," *Nederlands Tijdschrift voor Geneeskunde,* vol. 133 (1989): 1839–1844.

Monagle, R. N., "Relationship of birth outcome to health care provider." *American Journal of Obstetrics and Gynecology,* vol. 146 (1983): 870–871.

Pel, M., and P. E. Treffers, "The reliability of the result of the umbilical cord pH," *Journal of Perinatal Medicine,* vol. 11 (1983): 169–174.

Prechtl, H.F.R., and D. J. Beintema, "The neurological examination of the full term newborn infant," In: *Clinics in Developmental Medicine,* no 12 (London: Heinemann Medical Books, 1964).

Prentice, A., and T. Lind, "Fetal heart rate monitoring during labour: too frequent intervention, too little benefit?" *Lancet,* ii (1987): 1375–1377.

Rooks, J. P. et al, "Outcomes of care in birth centers: the National Birth Center Study," *New England Journal of Medicine,* vol. 321 (1989): 1804–1811.

Royal College of Obstetricians and Gynaecologists, Response to the Report of the House of Commons Health Committee on Maternity Services. London, 1992.

Springer, M. P., *Kwaliteit van het verloskundig handelen van huisartsen.* Thesis, University of Leiden, 1991.

Sykes, G. S. et al., "Do Apgar scores indicate asphyxia?" *Lancet,* i (1982): 494–496.

Tew, M., and S.M.J. Damstra-Wijmenga, "Safest birth attendants: recent Dutch evidence." *Midwifery,* vol 7 (1991): 55–63.

Treffers, P. E., D. van Alten, and M. Pel, "Condemnation of obstetric care in The Netherlands?" *American Journal of Obstetrics and Gynecology,* vol. 146 (1983): 871–872.

Treffers, P. E. et al. "Home births and minimal medical interventions," *Journal of the American Medical Association,* vol. 264 (1990): 2203–2208.

van Alten, D., M. Eskes, and P. E. Treffers, "Midwifery in the Netherlands; the Wormerveer study: selection, mode of delivery, perinatal mortality and infant morbidity," *British Journal of Obstetrics and Gynaecology,* vol. 96 (1989): 656–662.

Verloove-Vanhorick, S. P. et al., "Mortality in very preterm and very low-birth-weight infants according to place of birth and level of care," *Pediatrics*, vol. 81 (1988): 404–411.

Wolf, H., *Aspects of intrauterine growth and growth retardation.* Thesis, University of Amsterdam, 1991.

Ziekenfondsraad, *Verloskundige indicatielijst.* Amstelveen, 1987.

APPENDIX: LIST OF MEDICAL INDICATIONS (ABBREVIATED)

A = Primary care, delivery at home or in hospital
B = Consultation with the obstetrician
C = Secondary care by obstetrician in the hospital

1.1. Medical history

A. *Neurological diseases*

Epilepsy, subarachnoid hemorrhage, multiple sclerosis	B
Hernia nuclei pulposi (not developing during pregnancy)	A

B. *Medical disorders*

Tuberculosis	C
Bronchial asthma	B
Cardiac disorders	B
Thrombo-embolism	B
Clotting disorders	C
Nephropathy	B
Diabetes mellitus	C
Addison's disease, Cushing's disease	C
Hypothyroidism	B
Hyperthyroidism	C
Anemia, <6.0 mmol/L	B
Colitis ulcerosa, Crohn's disease	C

C. *Gynecological disorders*

Vaginal prolapse	B
Conization of the cervix	C
Myomectomy, subserous fibromyoma	A
Myomectomy, submucous or intramural fibromyoma	C
Vesicovaginal or rectovaginal fistula	C
Abnormal cervical cytology	A
In case of carcinoma	C
DES-exposed *in utero*	A

IUD *in situ*	A
Infertility	A
Pelvic fracture	B
D. *Miscellaneous*	
Use of hard drugs	C
Psychiatric disorders	B
1.2. Obstetrical history	
Rhesus sensitization	C
Pregnancy hypertension (in previous pregnancy)	A
Recurrent abortion in first trimester	A
Preterm delivery	B
Cervical incompetence	C
Abruptio placentae	C
Forcipal extraction or vacuum extraction	A
Caesarean section	C
Fetal growth retardation	C
Neonatal asphyxia	B
Fetal death	B
Neonatal death	B
Congenital malformation	B
Postpartum hemorrhage	B
Manual removal of placenta	B
Third-degree perineal tear	A
Puerperal psychosis	A
Symphysiolysis	A
Age of nulliparous woman over thirty-five years	B
Age of multiparous woman over forty years	B
Age under fifteen years	A
Grand multiparity	A
2. Abnormalities originating during the prenatal period	
Anemia, Hb <6.0 mmol/L	B
Pyelitis	A
Rubella, cytomegaly	A
Toxoplasmosis	C
Herpes simplex	B
Hepatitis Bs-Ag positive	A
Hernia nuclei pulposi, originating during pregnancy	B

Abnormality of cervical cytology	A
Use of hard drugs	C
Psychiatric disorders	B
Antenatal diagnosis (amniocentesis or chorion villus biopsy)	A
Suspicion of fetal malformation	B
Hypertension, diastolic greater than ninety-five	B
Proteinuria	B
Rhesus sensitization	C
Hemorrhage after twenty weeks	C
Abruptio placentae	C
Suspicion of fetal growth retardation	B or C
Postmaturity	C
Imminent preterm labor	C
Cervical incompetence	C
Multiple pregnancy	C
Malposition of the fetus	B or C
Disproportion in the third trimester	B
Fetal death	B or C

3. **Abnormalities during labor and delivery**

Malposition of the fetus	C
Signs of fetal distress	C
Ruptured membranes without contractions (> 24 hrs.)	C
Poor progress of labor or delivery	C
Abnormal hemorrhage during labor	C
Abruptio placentae	C
Vasa previa	C
Excessive hemorrhage during the third or fourth period	C
Retained placenta	C
Third-degree perineal tear	C
Complicated perineal tear	C

4. **Abnormalities in the puerperium** (for specialist care in hospital)

1. For the mother: vulval hematoma, serious puerperal infection, puerperal psychosis, thrombo-embolic disease

2. For the infant: growth retardation or preterm birth, cyanosis, hypothermia, serious congenital malformations, severe jaundice or jaundice in the first twenty-four hours.

6

How Safe Are Dutch Home Births?

Simone E. Buitendijk

INTRODUCTION

Even though the percentage of home births in the Netherlands has been declining steadily from the 1950s until the mid-1980s, it is still remarkably high compared to other Western countries. Since giving birth in the hospital has virtually become the standard everywhere else in the Western world, it should come as no surprise that the Dutch system of home births is under continuing scrutiny by numerous interested parties, Dutch and non-Dutch. Many people believe that the move towards hospital births in the United States and in most of Europe was based on evidence that giving birth in a hospital would increase the safety for woman and child. Not unexpectedly, therefore, the safety of home births is the very issue that is most hotly debated. Opponents of home births often use the argument that it involves higher risks for both mother and child than hospital births do. This debate is ongoing in most Western countries as well as in the Netherlands.

The Dutch are well aware of their exceptional position compared to other countries, and are motivated to monitor the quality of their system of pregnancy and birth care. Unfortunately, the issue of safety for home births is not likely to be resolved soon in a manner that will satisfy everyone. Many studies that have compared hospital to home birth have shortcomings in design. Since most of these shortcomings are inevitable, it is doubtful that conclusive evidence will ever be found.

In this chapter, an overview will be presented of existing literature on the risk or safety of delivering at home; the strengths and weaknesses of each

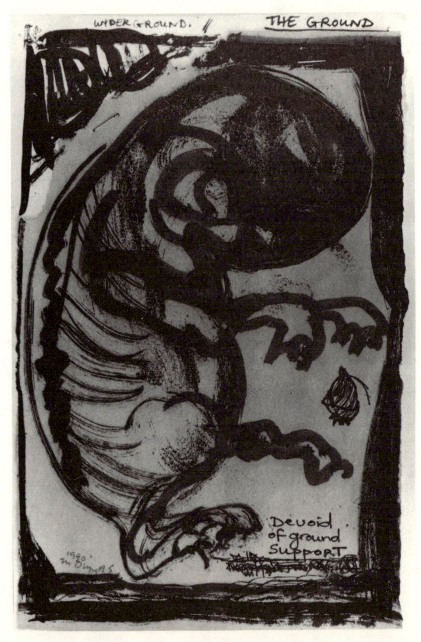

"Devoid of Ground Support," 1992 by Marlene Dumas. Photograph of illustration by Peter Cox. Used by permission of Marlene Dumas.

will be discussed, and some of the debate around the issue will be addressed. Finally, conclusions will be drawn with respect to the safety of home births and the possibilities for a pregnant woman's choice of place of birth.

THE IDEAL DESIGN TO STUDY THE RELATIVE SAFETY OF PLACE OF BIRTH

The best type of study to compare two different techniques or methods in health care is a randomized controlled trial (RCT), in which people are allocated by chance to two different treatments. The main advantage of this method is that, if the study is carried out well, the groups that are compared are truly equal. Factors that are hard to measure but may influence the outcome should be present in similar quantities in each group. Therefore, if differences in outcome are found, they are likely to have been caused by differences in the treatment studied. Ideally, an RCT into place of birth could be carried out by allocating half of a group of pregnant women to having the baby at home and half to having a hospital birth. Mortality and morbidity for the children and the women could subsequently be compared between the two groups. This type of approach would enable us to determine whether home and hospital births are equally safe, or whether one of the two is safer. In most of the present-day discussions, the burden of proof is on the advocates of home births, while it may be fruitful to ask whether hospital births are as safe as home births. An RCT could answer such a question. It is unlikely, however, that enough women nowadays would consent to being part of such a trial. Low-risk women who do have both options available to them would most likely be unwilling to participate in such a study, because the choice between home or hospital is often a highly motivated and conscious one. Women judged to be at higher risk, for obvious ethical reasons, could not be allocated to any but a hospital delivery. Furthermore, to study an outcome like mortality successfully, the number of women required to participate would have to be very large.

THE SITUATION IN PRACTICE

Most studies comparing different places of delivery are forced to compare groups of women that may not be equal in risk profile. Women delivering at home may be at higher or at lower risk than women delivering in the hospital (examples of both will be provided), which will lead to different outcomes for their children. Differences in mortality between countries may reflect population differences rather than variations in the quality of the obstetrical care systems. Nevertheless, the combined evidence can certainly be of value in determining whether the Dutch system is likely to be safe. There are pitfalls in using the perinatal mortality rate, one of the most frequently used outcome measures for studying the safety of home births. Examples will be discussed of instances where incorrect conclusions were drawn from studies that are based on this measure.

PERINATAL OR NEONATAL MORTALITY AS OUTCOME MEASURES

The perinatal mortality rate is defined as the number of late fetal and early neonatal deaths (deaths within the first week of life) per 1,000 live and still-births. The neonatal mortality rate is defined as the number of deaths within the first four weeks of life per 1,000 live births. Perinatal and neonatal mortality statistics are readily available in most countries, and have been used in many studies as indicators of the quality of care for a given place of delivery. Unfortunately, the use of these measures is not straightforward. To compare the perinatal mortality rate between countries or to study the trend in rate within countries as an indicator of the success of the obstetric care system can be very misleading.

First, individual countries use different definitions for perinatal mortality: they may define a live birth differently, since not all countries adhere to the definition suggested by the World Health Organization. A late fetal death may in some countries be defined as a death after nineteen weeks of gestation, while in others twenty-four or twenty-eight weeks is used as the cutoff point. The definition of early neonatal death can differ, depending on the number of hours that countries decide constitute a seven-day period (Golding and Butler, 1990). Second, recording may be incomplete. Personal variations in recording can exist within countries, depending on how obstetricians or midwives interpret official guidelines for reporting (Keirse, 1984), or underreporting may take place by region (Golding and Butler, 1990). This can result in different perinatal mortality rates for very comparable groups. To complicate matters even further, changes in definition or recording practices can occur over time, which can make some trend analyses quite unreliable.

Even with perfect definitions and recording practices, other factors than the quality of care, such as a change in general health of a population, may cause the perinatal mortality rate to change. These factors need to be taken into account before perinatal mortality trends can be used to draw conclusions about the quality of care. Another element that can make the comparison of perinatal mortality rates perilous is the rapid decline of such rates in most Western countries. As a result, the differences between countries are small, and modest fluctuations or changes can, for an individual country, mean the difference between being first or being fourth or fifth in the ranking order.

STUDIES USING TRENDS IN PERINATAL MORTALITY

Appropriate caution in interpreting perinatal mortality rates is not always practiced: The strong decline in perinatal mortality rates in many countries since the 1950s has frequently been linked to the increase in percentage of hospital births. In England in 1984, the chairperson of the Maternity Services Advisory Committee wrote: "The practice of delivering nearly all babies in the hospital has contributed to a dramatic reduction in stillbirths and neonatal deaths and to the avoidance of many child handicaps" (Campbell and Macfarlane, 1986). A number of English studies can be used to disprove this statement, one of which showed that the perinatal mortality rate declined in a similar fashion among hospital and home births (Barron, Thomson, and Philpis, 1977).

In 1978, D. Hoogendoorn, a Dutch author, graphically displayed the decline in perinatal mortality rate along with the increase in percentage of women delivering in the hospital between 1952 and 1975, corrected for maternal age and parity. He concluded that further hospitalization of birth would likely result in additional decrease in mortality (Hoogendoorn, 1978). Another Dutch study by Gerrit-Jan Kloosterman examined the shift in perinatal mortality rates and compared it to the shift to hospitalization in thirteen large Dutch cities during the early 1970s. This study concluded that there was no evidence of any relationship between the two factors (Kloosterman, 1978). In 1986, Hoogendoorn published another article comparing Dutch and Danish perinatal mortality trends (Hoogendoorn, 1986). The Dutch perinatal mortality rate had virtually stopped declining since the early 1980s, whereas the Danish rate was still showing improvement. The author offered as one possible explanation the fact that the Danes, in contrast to the Dutch, had since the 1970s almost completely shifted to hospital births. This article sparked a wide debate, the more since it received extensive press coverage. Hoogendoorn's opponents pointed out many other possible reasons for the contrast, such as differences in reporting, differences in population profile, and differences in prenatal screening policies that could have explained the differences in trends between Denmark and the Netherlands.

In contrast, Marjorie Tew, an English researcher, observed that during the period between 1969 and 1981, perinatal mortality fell least when the rate of hospitalization increased most. She concluded that the trend in declining mortality rates would have been more favorable had hospitalization of birth taken place at a slower rate (Tew, 1986).

However, the trend to increasing hospitalization of births cannot be causally linked to the trend in mortality rates. Such findings cannot prove that hospitalization was responsible for speeding up or slowing down the decline in perinatal mortality rates. Conclusions like these often seem to stem from preconceived notions for which the author tries to find scientific evidence. They should not be taken at face value.

STUDIES COMPARING MORTALITY RATES IN HOME AND HOSPITAL BIRTHS

Using perinatal mortality to compare the quality of home versus hospital deliveries requires a large number of women in both groups because of the low mortality rates. Many of the studies do not have enough subjects, and as a result, the similarity in mortality rates between the two groups can reflect equal safety as well as lack of statistical power to find a truly existing difference.

When perinatal mortality figures are used to evaluate the safety of home births within countries, special attention needs to be paid to the fact that a percentage of women who deliver at home may not have planned to do so. Since this subgroup is at higher risk of adverse outcomes, the result will be an increase in the mortality rate for home births compared to those taking place in the hospital. If this is the case, different mortality rates need not necessarily reflect different effectiveness of care. A number of observational studies from different countries have compared mortality rates in home versus hospital births. One retrospective study from the 1970s from North Carolina, showed that home deliveries had a two times higher risk of neonatal mortality than hospital deliveries (Schramm et al., 1987). However, after allowance was made for planned and unplanned home births, a different picture emerged. Planned home births had a much lower risk than hospital births, whereas unplanned home births had a ten times higher risk than hospital births. Another U.S. study showed that unplanned home births had twenty times the risk of neonatal mortality as planned home births (Burnett et al., 1980). A study of home births in England and Wales showed that women with planned home births had the lowest mortality rate (4.1 per 1,000), whereas the group whose delivery had been booked in the hospital but occurred at home had a risk that was almost seventeen times higher, namely sixty-seven per 1,000. The highest rate occurred in home births that had not been booked at either place. The mortality was almost fifty times higher than in the planned home birth group, 197 per 1,000. Although these finding cannot prove the safety of planned home births, they do illustrate that it is incorrect to compare crude rates for home and hospital births without taking the possibility of selection into account.

Although place of delivery seems a clearly defined measure for studying mortality rates, grouping women who do not give birth in the place they had planned to may not be straightforward. If a complication arises that prompts a hospital delivery when a home delivery was planned, the (possibly complicated) birth will count as a hospital birth. Similarly, when a woman goes into preterm labor so fast that she cannot reach the hospital in time, this birth will be counted as a home birth. The issue of whether data should be analyzed by intended or actual place of delivery has not yet been answered satisfactorily. To measure adverse effects of obstetrical interventions in women originally booked for home deliveries, the analysis should be carried out by actual place of birth (Tew, 1978). However, if antenatal care is different in women booked for a home or a hospital birth so that it can influence the outcome of the pregnancy, an analysis by intended place of delivery should be carried out (Murphy et al., 1984). The main problem in using actual place of delivery is that purposeful selection for transfer to a hospital of women who experience some kind of complication during pregnancy or delivery will increase the likelihood of adverse outcomes in the hospital group. Some unfavorable outcomes will thus be included in the hospital delivery group, even though a delivery began at home. This will lower the rate of complications in the home birth group. Thus, analyses by intended place of delivery, rather than actual place, tend to decrease the estimated perinatal mortality rate for hospital births and increase the rate for home births (Campbell and MacFarlane, 1986). If information on intended as well as actual place of delivery is available (which is not always the case), it may be worthwhile to use both measures and compare the results while keeping in mind the limitations involved in both approaches.

Trends in crude mortality in home births compared to hospital births may prove misleading during periods when deliveries increasingly take place in the hospital. The shift will especially take place in the group of women who in the past had home deliveries that were planned. Home deliveries for young teenagers who have made no delivery arrangements or for women who go into labor early and unexpectedly will continue at the same rate. The shift will result in a higher proportion of unplanned home births and, consequently, shows an increased mortality rate for home births (Campbell et al., 1982; Murphy et al., 1984). Thus, the increase in mortality rates in home births cannot be used as evidence for their decreasing safety.

Similarly, the use of retrospectively adjusted data to show that hospital interventions make births unsafe may not be justified. Tew used British and Dutch perinatal mortality data to conclude just that (Tew, 1986). After retrospectively adjusting for a number of known risk factors, such as age, parity, birth weight, and an antenatal and labor prediction score, she found that the mortality rates in hospital births were still significantly higher than those in home births. She argued that this difference could not have been explained by the greater proportion at risk in the hospital group and concluded that the very obstetric interventions used to make birth safer had had the opposite effect. Although her arguments may seem reasonable, it is unclear whether her method of statistically controlling for certain factors successfully dealt with unknown biases. Such biases may be introduced because of the subtle selection processes that may influence a woman's choice for home or hospital delivery. There is indeed some evidence that even when statistical adjustment is based on a large amount of descriptive data, this approach can still be seriously misleading (Murphy et al., 1984).

Tew found confirmation for her theories in the Dutch National Obstetrics Database (LVR). In 1986, the perinatal mortality rate for babies of short gestation was 46.4 for obstetricians compared to 12.6 for midwives. For full-term births, the rates are 8.1 and 0.8, respectively (Tew, 1990). Although I agree with Tew that it is unlikely these rates are purely accidental, I do not believe they prove that midwives provide women with safer births. It is very likely that preterm births under midwives' care are of a very different nature than those under the supervision of obstetricians. This is certainly the case for full-term births, since the entire Dutch system of obstetrics is based on a selection system for risk. Similar figures for perinatal mortality in births attended by Dutch midwives and obstetricians exist for 1988: Mortality of all births after sixteen weeks of pregnancy was twenty-three times higher in the babies delivered under the care of obstetricians (thirty per 1,000) than in those delivered by midwives (1.3 per 1,000). For term births only, these figures were six per 1,000 and one per 1,000, respectively (SIG-jaarboek, 1992). These figures show that the system works well and that midwives most likely do an excellent job selecting and providing care to women at low risk. They do not show that obstetricians' interventions make births unsafe or that midwives provide better care than obstetricians.

WHICH DATA CAN BE USED? THE COMBINED EVIDENCE

It is possible, however, to draw some conclusions about the safety of home births from available data, despite the difficulties in interpreting them. Although unknown differences in risk profile, even in low-risk women, may have influenced outcomes in the studies to be discussed, and some only include a small number of women, their conclusions all point in the same direction. Given the unavailability of randomized trials, these studies are the only evidence we can presently use.

With the exception of Tew's investigation (Tew, 1986), showing a lower risk of complications for out-of-hospital births, most studies reflect no difference in adverse outcomes or risk for the baby between home and hospital deliveries, or they show a higher risk that disappears for the low-risk subgroup with trained birth attendants present.

Lewis E. Mehl studied over 1,100 women in the United States, matched for age, education, obstetric risk factors, and socio-economic status. No differences in mortality or neurological impairment were found between those intending to give birth at home and those who chose to go to a hospital (Mehl et al., 1977). A small prospective study in England compared about 200 low-risk home births to a similar number of low-risk hospital births and showed no perinatal deaths in either group (Shearer, 1985). Claude Burnett, in his study of 1,296 U.S. home births, found no difference in neonatal mortality rate when low-risk home births were compared to hospital births of similar birth weight babies (Burnett et al., 1980). Another study carried out in the United States looked at 3,067 planned home births and compared them to hospital births. After adjustment had been made for race, age of the mother, and birth weight, the neonatal mortality rate was higher than in hospital births. This difference, however, was found only in the group of women whose births had not been attended by a trained midwife (Schramm et al., 1987). In an Australian study of 800 planned home births, a higher perinatal mortality rate was found for women delivering at home. There was evidence, however, that high-risk women had been included in the home birth group and that difficulties had arisen with transport to the hospital (Crotty et al., 1990). A study into cerebral palsy rates in children born in Northern England between 1960 and 1975 showed lower rates among children born at home than in the hospital, after accounting for differences in birth weight distribution (Jarvis, Holloway, and Hey, 1985).

Most Dutch studies into the rate of complications in home births differ from the studies mentioned above: the selection system resulted in substantially lower risk for women delivering at home than those delivering in the hospital. The perinatal mortality rate in Dutch home births, as well as the rate of other adverse outcomes, is almost by definition substantially lower than in the entire group of (low- and high-risk) hospital births (van Alten, Eskes, and Treffers, 1989; Eskes, Knuist, and van Alten, 1987; Knuist, Eskes, and van Alten, 1987; Berghs and Spanjaards, 1988). The issue of how successful this screening system is will be dealt with by Pieter E. Treffers elsewhere in this volume. A study by G.A.H. Berghs comparing perinatal outcomes in low-risk Dutch women delivered by midwives (these deliveries can take place at home or in the hospital) to low-risk women delivered by obstetricians showed equal rates of adverse neurological outcomes between the two groups (Berghs and Spanjaards, 1988). Neurological outcomes are often considered to be sensitive measures for problems stemming from prolonged labor and lack of oxygen during delivery (Dennis and Chalmers, 1981).

These comparisons suggest that for low-risk women who have a well-trained attendant present at birth, outcomes of home births are similar to those of hospital births. These data cannot "prove" that home births are safe, since subtle differences in characteristics between low-risk women preferring home or hospital as their site of birth may influence the likelihood of adverse outcomes. The Berghs study also showed that women delivering under the care of an obstetrician for whom no medical or obstetrical indication existed were more likely to have a lower educational level and to smoke and drink during pregnancy (Berghs and Spanjaards, 1988). Evidence from a study by Treffers shows that women in rural areas are much more likely to have home births than women in urban areas (Treffers and Laan, 1986). These differences are so large that they cannot be accounted for simply because of different obstetric risk profiles; they are very likely related to cultural differences as well as differences in geographical proximity to obstetric hospitals. Subtle differences that are difficult to measure with formal scoring systems, but may result in differences in risk profile and outcome may also play a part. Many other studies have shown that women planning a home birth may be of different socio-economic status than those having a hospital birth (Schneider, 1986; Schramm et al., 1987; Crotty et al., 1990; Kleiverda et al., 1990; Anderson and Greener, 1990).

Murphy et al. studied over 44,000 English women who gave birth between

1970 and 1979 (Murphy et al., 1984). The authors found that both mortality and morbidity (respiratory problems, among others) in babies born at home were low compared to those in the population at large.

One of the best studies dealing with the safety of home births is a study by Treffers in the Netherlands comparing perinatal mortality rates and the percentage of hospital deliveries in the eleven Dutch provinces (Treffers and Laan, 1986). Its conclusions add to the evidence derived from the studies discussed before. Hospitalization at delivery varied from 49.2 percent to 75.5 percent among provinces, but no relationship with perinatal mortality could be found. Similarly, perinatal mortality was not lower in large cities, where the percentage of hospital deliveries was high, compared to small towns and villages where, traditionally, births are more likely to take place at home. When cities with more than 100,000 inhabitants were compared to small towns, no relationship could be found between the perinatal mortality rate and the degree of hospitalization at birth (which varied from 50.5 percent to 95.7 percent from urban center to urban center). It is unlikely that differences in notification practices or population profiles can account for the absence of an effect of hospitalization rate on mortality. Further, the numbers of births studied were large enough to enable detection of a moderate difference in rates if it had been present. These findings lend further support to the theory that within a good selection system, home births do not result in higher perinatal mortality than hospital births.

DIFFERENCES IN INTERVENTION RATES BETWEEN HOME AND HOSPITAL BIRTHS

From all the studies comparing home and hospital deliveries, large differences in obstetric intervention rates between the two groups emerge, even when women with similar obstetric risk profiles are compared. One English study showed an induction rate of 19 percent in the low-risk hospital group, compared to 8 percent in the group of women booked for delivery at home. It also found a higher rate of episiotomy and second-degree tears in the hospital birth group (Shearer, 1985). Another study showed lower risks of induction, epidural anesthesia, episiotomy, and Caesarean section in the group of women who planned their labor at home (Crotty et al., 1990). This is in accordance with data suggesting that when the technology level of the hospital where low-risk women give birth increases, so does the use of intervention procedures for childbirth (Albers and Katz, 1991). A study by Mehl in the United States comparing groups of women with similar risk factors found that the rate of episiotomy was five times higher among the hospital group than among the home birth group (Mehl et al., 1977). Berghs, who studied a low-risk obstetrical population in the Netherlands, showed that obstetricians had much higher rates of interventions compared to midwives and general practitioners. They were more likely to use oxytocin, amniotomy, anesthesia, and episiotomies (Berghs and Spanjaards, 1988). These findings suggest an increased risk of interventions for low-risk women delivering in the hospital, along with increased iatrogenic risk.

ARE HOME BIRTHS SAFE?

The shift towards hospital births has not been the cause of the decline in perinatal mortality rates. Based on all the available evidence, there is no indication that home births are not safe for low-risk pregnancies or that hospital births are intrinsically safer. Dutch as well as international studies show that women can be successfully screened for risk factors and that a valid definition of low risk can indeed be made. There is no evidence that perinatal outcome can be improved if all women deliver in the hospital.

A successful system of home births will be possible only if appropriate screening for risk can take place, care by an obstetrician is available if needed, and if a system of postpartum home care is in place. In the Netherlands, the presence of highly skilled midwives, a well-developed system of referral, cooperation among the professional groups taking care of pregnant women, and an organized program of professional home care after delivery permit the system of home births to work.

THE ISSUE OF CHOICE

Among women with low-risk pregnancies, the issue of their babies' safety should not affect their choice between home or hospital delivery. Rather, the choice (if available) should be strongly guided by personal preference only. In Dutch and international surveys of women who had experienced both home and hospital deliveries, the majority of women rated the home delivery as more satisfying (Alment et al., 1967; Fleury, 1967; Goldthorp and Richman, 1974; O'Brien, 1978; Kleiverda et al., 1990). In countries where home births are rare, some researchers believe that women may prefer home birth because of a previous unpleasant experience with hospital delivery (Fraser, 1983). Gunilla Kleiverda shows, however, that when both options are available, even women who are pregnant for the first time are able to express very clearly their preference for place of birth (Kleiverda et al., 1990). Of a group of 170 low-risk women experiencing their first pregnancies, only twenty-five were in doubt about where they wanted to have their baby. When interviewed during their eighteenth week of pregnancy, 100 of the women who had made up their minds preferred birth at home, and forty-five wanted to deliver in the hospital. Educational level, anxiety concerning possible complications, and attitudes towards female roles were factors that influenced the choice. After delivery, home births were assessed as more positive than hospital births. Most of the women said they preferred to have their next baby also in the same place. This preference was not influenced by the actual events encountered during the last delivery. Even in cases where intrapartum referrals from home to the hospital had taken place, the majority of women said they would opt for a home birth again. This finding is in accordance with results of a study in England (Caplan and Madeley, 1985) showing that around 90 percent of women who had either successfully completed a home birth or a hospital birth wanted to give birth in the same place again.

CONCLUSIONS

Since there is no scientific basis to advocate the use of hospital procedures for all women giving birth, and since there is evidence that when low-risk women plan to deliver in the hospital the risk of all types of obstetrical interventions is much higher than when they plan to have their deliveries at home, it seems that women should be given the choice of place of delivery. Available evidence suggests that when given this choice, many women in the Netherlands and other countries have strong opinions about where they want to have their babies.

In the United Kingdom, where the percentage of home births has been declining steadily since the beginning of this century, and presently births almost completely take place in the hospital, a Health Committee of the House of Commons has recently addressed the very issue of availability of options to pregnant women (Health Committee, 1992). Their conclusion, based on expert testimonies and review of the literature is that "the policy of encouraging all women to give birth in the hospital cannot be justified on grounds of safety.... The choices of a home birth or a hospital birth have been withdrawn from the majority of women in this country. For most women there is no choice. This does not appear to be in accordance with their wishes." Based on its conclusions, the committee goes on to make recommendations for changes that may enable women to gain more control over the birth process and to have low-technology options for place of birth available to them.

There is no evidence that the Dutch system of care for pregnant women can be improved by increasing medicalization of birth. Moreover, the data suggest that Dutch women are happy with the options they have. Experience from other countries, where home births have become almost nonexistent (sometimes rather rapidly), should motivate the Dutch to preserve and defend their system carefully, without abandoning healthy criticism of aspects that can be improved.

REFERENCES

Albers, Leah L., and Vern L. Katz, "Birth setting for low-risk pregnancies. An analysis of the current literature," *Journal of Nurse-Midwifery* 36 (1991): 215–220.
Alment, E.A.J., A. Barr, M. Reid, and J.J.A. Reid, "Normal confinement: a domiciliary and hospital study," *British Medical Journal* ii (1967): 530–535.

Anderson, Rondi, and Deborah Greener, "A descriptive analysis of home births attended by CNMs in two nurse-midwifery services," *Journal of Nurse-Midwifery* 36 (1990): 95-103.

Barron, S. L., A. M. Thomson, and P. R. Philpis, "Hospital and hospital confinement in Newcastle upon Tyne 1960-69," *British Journal of Obstetrics and Gynaecology* 84 (1977): 401-411.

Berghs, G.A.H., and E.W.M. Spanjaards, *"De Normale Zwangerschap: Bevalling en Beleid,"* Dissertation. Nijmegen, 1988.

Burnett, Claude A., James A. Jones, Judith Rooks, Chong Hwa Chen, Carl W. Tyler, and C. Arden Miller, "Home delivery and neonatal mortality in North Carolina," *Journal of the American Medical Association* 244 (1980): 2741-2745.

Campbell, Rona, Isobel MacDonald Davies, Alison Macfarlane, and Valerie Beral, "Home births in England and Wales, 1979: perinatal mortality according to intended place of delivery," *British Medical Journal* 289 (1982): 721-724.

Campbell, Rona, and Alison Macfarlane, "Place of delivery: A review," *British Journal of Obstetrics and Gynaecology* 93 (1986): 675-683.

Caplan, M., and R. J. Madeley, "Home deliveries in Nottingham 1980-81," *Public Health* 99 (1985): 307-313.

Crotty, Maria, Andrew T. Ramsey, Rosemary Smart, and Annabelle Chan, "Planned homebirths in South Australia 1976-1987," *Medical Journal of Australia* 153 (1990): 664-671.

Dennis, J., and I. Chalmers, "Very early neonatal seizure rate: a possible epidemiological indicator of the quality of perinatal care," in *Aspects of Perinatal Morbidity*, Huisjes H. J. (ed.) (Groningen: Veenstra Visser Offset, 1981).

Eskes, M., M. Knuist, and D. van Alten, "Neurologisch Onderzoek bij Pasgeborenen in een Verloskundigen Praktijk," *Nederlands Tijdschrift voor Geneeskunde* 131 (1987): 1040-1043.

Fleury, P. M., *Maternity Care. Mothers' Experience of Childbirth.* (London: Allen and Unwin, 1967).

Fraser, C. M., "Selected perinatal procedures. Scientific basis for use and psychological effects," *Acta Obstetrics and Gynecology Scandinavica, Supplement* 117 (1983): 11-12.

Golding, Jean, and N. R. Butler, "Studies of perinatal mortality: contrasts and contradictions," in *Social and Biological Effects on Perinatal Mortality*, Volume III: Perinatal Analysis. Report on an International Comparative Study Sponsored by the World Health Organization. Golding, J. (ed.) (Bristol: University of Bristol Printing Unit, 1990).

Goldthorp, W. O., and J. Richman, "Maternal attitudes to unintended home confinement. A case study of the effects of the hospital strike upon domiciliary confinements," *Practitioner* 212 (1974): 845-853.

Health Committee, Second report, *Maternity Services*, House of Commons Session 1991-92, Volume I. London: HMSO, 1992.

Hoogendoorn, D., "De Relatie Tussen de Hoogte van de Perinatale Sterfte en de Plaats van de Bevalling: Thuis, Dan Wel in het Ziekenhuis," *Nederlands Tijdschrift voor Geneeskunde* 122 (1978): 1171-1184.

Hoogendoorn, D., "Indrukwekkende en Tegelijk Teleurstellende Daling van de

Perinatale Sterfte in Nederland," *Nederlands Tijdschrift voor Geneeskunde* 130 (1986): 1436–1440.

Jarvis, S. N., J. S. Holloway, and E. Hey, "Increase in cerebral palsy in normal birth-weight babies," *Archives of Disease in Childhood* 60 (1985): 113–1121.

Keirse, Marc J.N.C., "Perinatal mortality rates do not contain what they purport to contain," *Lancet* i (1984): 1166–1168.

Kleiverda, Gunilla, A. M. Steen, Ingerlise Andersen, P. E. Treffers, and E. Everaerd, "Place of delivery in the Netherlands: maternal motives and background variables related to preferences for home or hospital confinement," *European Journal of Obstetrics, Gynaecology and Reproductive Biology* 36 (1990): 1–9.

Kloosterman, G. J., "De Nederlandse Verloskunde op de Tweesprong," *Nederlands Tijdschrift voor Geneeskunde* 122 (1978): 1161–1171.

Knuist, M., M. Eskes, and D. van Alten, "De pH van het Arteriële Navelstrengbloed van Pasgeborene bij door Vroedvrouwen Geleide Bevallingen," *Nederlands Tijdschrift voor Geneeskunde* 131 (1987): 362–365.

Mehl, Lewis E., Gail H. Peterson, Michael Whitt, and Warren E. Hawes, "Outcomes of elective home births: a series of 1,146 cases," *Journal of Reproductive Medicine* 19 (1977): 281–290.

Murphy, J. F., Marjorie Dauncey, O. P. Gray, and I. Chalmers, "Planned and unplanned deliveries at home: implications of a changing ratio," *British Medical Journal* 288 (1984): 1429–1432.

O'Brien, M. "Home and hospital confinement: comparison of the experiences of mothers having home and hospital confinements," *J. Roy. Coll. Gen. Pract.* 28 (1978): 460–466.

Schneider, Dona, "Planned out-of-hospital births. New Jersey, 1978–1980," *Social Science Medicine* 23 (1986): 1011–1015.

Schramm, Wayne F., Diane E. Barnes, and Janice M. Bakewell, "Neonatal mortality in Missouri home births, 1978–84," *American Journal of Public Health* 77 (1987): 930–935.

Shearer, J.M.L. "Five year prospective survey of risk of booking for a home birth in Essex," *British Medical Journal* 291 (1985): 1478–1480.

SIG (Stichting Informatiecentrum Gezondheidszorg), "Jaarboek LVR-1 en LVR-2 1988," Utrecht: SIG, 1992.

Tew, Marjorie, "Intended place of delivery and perinatal outcome (letter)," *British Medical Journal* 91 (1978): 1139–1140.

Tew, Marjorie, "Do obstetric intranatal interventions make birth safer?" *British Journal of Obstetrics and Gynaecology* 93 (1986): 659–674.

Tew, Marjorie, *Safer Childbirth? A Critical History of Maternity Care*, Tew. M. (ed.) (London, New York, Tokyo, Melbourne, Madras: Chapman and Hall, 1990): 266–270.

Treffers, P. E., and R. Laan, "Regional perinatal mortality and regional hospitalization at delivery in the Netherlands," *British Journal of Obstetrics and Gynaecology* 93 (1986): 690–693.

van Alten, D., M. Eskes, and P. E. Treffers, "Midwifery in the Netherlands; the Wormerveer study; selection mode of delivery, perinatal mortality and infant morbidity," *British Journal of Obstetrics and Gynaecology* 96 (1989): 656–662.

7

The Impact of Medical-Technological Developments on Midwifery in the Netherlands

Tjeerd Tymstra

INTRODUCTION

The midwife occupies a central position in the Dutch health service, but she may assist only in normal physiological pregnancies. For pregnancies that may put mother or child at risk, the role of technology is becoming increasingly important. Beyond technology to assist the birth process, there is also technology to examine and safeguard mother and fetus. For instance, an increasing number of early diagnostic tests for congenital abnormalities are becoming available. Such technologies are often difficult to incorporate into midwifery practice, however. They have a strongly medicalizing effect, which leads to pregnant women becoming more and more dependent on the medical system. Although such dependency is not unusual in many Western countries, medicalization goes counter to the existing care pattern in the Netherlands, which is based on the natural character of pregnancy and delivery. For the Dutch midwife, these new technologies create an area of tension. In this chapter, we elaborate on these problems.

ULTRASOUND TECHNOLOGY

Ultrasonics have made it possible to obtain sharper and clearer pictures of the fetus inside the uterus. In many Western countries, ultrasound is now widely used during pregnancy, and this has become the case in the Netherlands as well. Those in favor of ultrasound point out that the technology provides insight into whether a pregnancy is vital, the gestational age of the

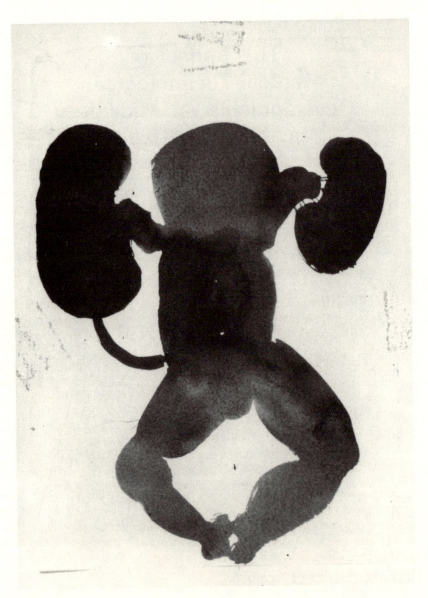

"Life Before Birth" (watercolor) by Malene Dumas. Used by permission of Marlene Dumas.

fetus can be accurately predicted, and the diagnosis of multiple pregnancies is improved. Ultrasound also has a very strong attraction for the pregnant woman and her partner: people enjoy being able to see pictures of their unborn child (and being able to take them home), and it can even lead to stronger bonds between the mother and child because it enables the woman to see her child.

As with every medical technology, however, there are also a number of disadvantages and objections: the financial cost, anxiety and uncertainty, overtreatment, and the possibility of iatrogenic damage. Probably the most important objection to ultrasound is that it leads to the technicalization and medicalization of pregnancy. Ultrasound examination contributes to a greater number of pregnant women being placed under medical supervision, in direct opposition to the natural character of pregnancy. In other words, it seriously affects the basic character of the Dutch approach to pregnancy, which is one of the major reasons why many Dutch midwives hesitate to use ultrasound. They have engaged in debates about whether ultrasound scanning should be encouraged, and if so, whether they should learn and carry out the technical procedures themselves. Those in favor argue that it is important for midwives to be able to use ultrasound and for its use to take place within midwifery practice.

One of the strongest proponents of this view is P.A.O.M. de Reu,[1] a male midwife (about 3 percent of Dutch midwives are males), who argues that midwives must avoid the risk of a calamity during pregnancy and (home) delivery, and must therefore make use of preventive technologies. He says, "We as midwives should be much better informed about the state of health, the 'quality' of the pregnancy product, than for example an obstetrician in one of the best equipped hospitals in the United States; from this point of view, it is my opinion that routine ultrasound examination during pregnancy is advisable at the very least." He adds, "An attitude of rejection toward ultrasound can mean the end of the independence of our careers." Nor can the importance of ultrasound to the status and prestige of the midwife be ignored, points out de Reu.

Some midwives undermine their own position by first indicating the disadvantages and risks of delivering at home, and then going on to say that the at-risk group could be reduced considerably through ultrasound examination.[2] It has also been postulated that by performing the ultrasound scan themselves, the midwives would lose fewer patients to the obstetricians.[3] But there are also many Dutch midwives who would like to restrict the use of ultrasound because they do not see any advantages to the routine use of this technology,[4] and the Dutch Organization of Midwives itself has considerable reservations regarding the use of ultrasound.

It is impossible to imagine obstetrics today without ultrasound. Over the past few years, more and more pregnant women have been undergoing this technique, even under the supervision of a midwife (in 1991, 10 percent of the midwife practices had ultrasound technology). In addition, because the technology has been improved and the images of the fetus are clearer, the technique is applied to an increasing extent to those at risk for congenital abnormalities. The issue is: do all pregnant women need to undergo such an examination?[5] Obviously, this would have great consequences for Dutch obstetrics.

CONGENITAL ABNORMALITIES

Only in the last few decades has medical care during pregnancy gone beyond the role of watching that a delivery ran its proper course. The new role was made possible by technologies that can provide information about the fetus inside the uterus (chromosomal investigation). Subsequently, in many countries, amniocentesis and chorionic villi sampling were offered to older pregnant women to determine if the fetus had a chromosomal abnormality. In the Netherlands, too, these tests have been available for more than twenty years. In 1985, the age limit for amniocentesis or chorionic villi sampling was lowered from thirty-eight to thirty-six (i.e., at eighteen weeks of pregnancy, the woman must be at least thirty-six years old). Younger pregnant women are not eligible for these tests, even if they are prepared to pay for them themselves. Contrary to its European neighbors, the Netherlands has always pursued a uniform central policy in this field.

In this country, in 1988, 51 percent of the pregnant women thirty-six years or older had amniocentesis or chorionic villi sampling.[6] Studies have shown that the most important reasons for refusing such prenatal diagnostics include moral objections to the test (by those who are against abortion), fear of miscarriage or fetal damage, and "acceptance" that the child may be handicapped (God's will).[7] Moreover, the same study revealed that some of the women were not aware or had not been told that the tests were available. This raises the question of how doctors and midwives inform older pregnant women about the possibilities of prenatal diagnosis. In the early 1980s, a pilot study on this topic was carried out in the northern provinces of the Netherlands by interviewing older mothers about their experiences (women who had made use of prenatal diagnosis as well as those who had not). One of the women who had delivered a healthy baby a few months prior to the study told us: "I was 38 years old and brought the subject to the attention of the midwife myself. She was against me having amniocentesis, because no one in my family had any abnormalities. So I didn't have the test."

Prenatal diagnosis makes it possible to prevent the birth of a handicapped child. However, amniocentesis and chorionic villi sampling also entail a great deal of stress and anxiety, and may lead to iatrogenic damage (miscarriage). As the age limit for these tests is lowered, the disadvantages of the tests begin to outweigh the advantages (a forty-year-old woman runs a 1:100 risk of having a child with Down's syndrome; at thirty-six the risk is 1:250). Although the midwife mentioned above may have wished to reassure her client by sparing her the stress of prenatal diagnosis, the woman was not reassured at all. She said, "My husband and I never agreed with the midwife, and we were under a lot of stress in the last few months. Luckily it all turned out well in the end."

Some years ago, legal proceedings were taken against a Dutch obstetrician who had not informed an older pregnant woman adequately of the possibility of prenatal diagnosis (she delivered a child with Down's syndrome). He was reprimanded: it is the duty of all health professionals to inform pregnant women of the possibility of amniocentesis and chorionic villi sampling. Dutch midwives are also obliged to follow this policy, and lowering the age limit for the tests will mean that many more pregnant women will be confronted by prenatal diagnosis. Further, with increasingly more tests being developed to detect fetal abnormalities, how are midwives supposed to deal with the new ones? Should they also be made available?

SERUM TESTS

By analyzing the alpha-fetoprotein level (AFP) in amniotic fluid, it is possible to determine whether the fetus has a neural tube defect. At the end of the 1970s, it became clear that AFP analysis of maternal serum could help to predict whether the fetus had spina bifida or craniofenestria (a high serum AFP level is indicative of an increased risk for these abnormalities). Serum tests are fairly simple to perform and are inexpensive, which makes such tests suitable for mass-screening programs. By detecting the pregnant women who have a raised serum AFP level and offering them further tests (ultrasound, amniocentesis), it will be possible to trace a large proportion of fetuses with a neural tube defect at an early stage. In a number of countries (Great Britain, Sweden, the United States), mass-screening programs for serum AFP are already under way. In the Netherlands, policy makers have been very reluctant to offer this test, fearing it might give rise to many false-positive results (the test initially suggests abnormality, which may subsequently be negative, suggesting normality), resulting in unnecessary anxiety for many women. In 1989, the Dutch minister of health rejected mass serum AFP screening, but the test may be carried out in individual cases.

Nevertheless, some Dutch teaching hospitals have been offering the serum AFP test to pregnant women for many years, and it is gradually becoming more widely known among health professionals and the general public. An increasing number of pregnant women request serum AFP analysis, leading to many more serum AFP tests being conducted, especially in the vicinity of university centers. Thus, despite rejection by the government, strong diffusion of this technology is taking place.

It is clear that the existence of the diagnostic procedures has consequences for Dutch midwives. In 1991, a pilot study investigated how some Dutch midwives in the north of the country felt about the tests. One midwife was very positive about serum AFP analysis. In his practice (he is a man-midwife), the test led to the early detection of a serious congenital abnormality. Since then, he has been informing all the pregnant women in his practice about the existence of serum AFP analysis ("I have experienced what it means first hand and therefore advise people to use it"). The interviews with other midwives, however, showed that this attitude is not at all representative. It is clear that many midwives are not in favor of serum AFP screening: it causes pregnant women a great deal of anxiety and undermines "the natural character" of being pregnant.

NEW DEVELOPMENTS

Medical science never stands still, and it has now become clear that a low serum AFP level also has predictive value: it means that the pregnant woman runs a higher risk of delivering a child with a chromosomal abnormality. There are other new and relatively simple testing methods for detecting congenital abnormalities as well: recent studies have shown that the serum concentration of estriol and human chorionic gonadotropin are also predictors of chromosomal abnormalities in the fetus. All these blood tests are suitable for mass screening of pregnant women, which, when combined with age adjustments, make it possible to detect 60 percent of chromosomal abnormalities.[8] This percentage is considerably higher than that obtained using only the existing age-selection criteria, but the Dutch government has reservations about mass screening. At the end of 1991, the Dutch minister of health openly expressed opposition against the application of mass screening for these serum markers.

At some Dutch teaching hospitals, experiments are carried out with the new serum markers, which can lead to a situation in which a normal thirty-year-old pregnant woman can be told, "The results of the serum test show that your risk of having a child with Down's syndrome is not 1:1,000, which is normal for your age, but 1:250" (the same risk as for a normal thirty-six-year-old pregnant woman). At the Groningen teaching hospital, we performed a study examining how women who had been told on the basis of the serum test that they ran an increased risk of delivering a child with Down's syndrome coped with this information. For this purpose, interviews were conducted with twenty younger pregnant women who had undergone a serum test at the University Hospital Groningen. We found that the participants were not very well informed about the meaning of the serum test. Those who received the news that the blood test had indicated an increased risk of delivering a child with Down's syndrome found it very stressful. The women did not think in terms of "now I run a greater risk," but were more or less convinced that "there is something wrong with my baby." Consequently, the majority of women were determined to undergo amniocentesis to be certain ("I can't get through these nine months with such a feeling of uncertainty; I've got to know for sure whether there is anything wrong").[9]

It is not possible to stop medical technological developments; more techniques are becoming available that will benefit some, but may present problems for others or for society as a whole. Important developments have been made in the area of fetal surgery (operating or treating the fetus inside the uterus). If pregnant women are offered an ultrasound scan to detect a treatable fetal abnormality, many would wish to undergo the scan. This is clear from a study conducted on a group of women from the Groningen teaching hospital who had had their first baby a few months previously. We presented them with the following situation: Of all the babies born in the Netherlands, 1 in 1,500 has a serious kidney disease. This disease often arises during pregnancy: the fetus' urethra is too narrow (the duct by which urine is discharged from the bladder), so the urine flows back towards the kidneys. With the aid of ultrasound scanning, this abnormality can be detected between the twenty-first and twenty-sixth week of pregnancy. If this abnormality is detected during pregnancy, then it is possible, either during pregnancy or directly after delivery, to perform an operation to prevent kidney damage. Would you undergo such a test during a future pregnancy if you were offered the opportunity? Eighty-seven percent of the women said that they would undergo the test, 10 percent would not, and 3 percent were not sure.[10] Pregnant women find it very difficult to resist such diagnostic tests: they do not want to feel responsible for the abnormality or suffering of their child. Such diagnostic tests therefore have a very imperative character.

CHOICE-GIVING TECHNOLOGIES

An increasing number of medical technologies are associated with choices and risks. The term choice-giving technology is particularly applicable to prenatal diagnosis. This gives rise to the question of how people cope with such information. Over the past few years, there have been a number of studies investigating this topic. A group of young mothers were asked if they would take their newborn babies to a screening clinic for twenty-four hours to undergo tests for the early detection (and adequate treatment) of a serious illness known to occur in 1 in 90,000 cases. Over one-third (38 percent) of the respondents said they would participate, 28 percent were undecided, and the rest said they would not participate. The following question was asked of a group of blood donors: Imagine you underwent a medical procedure with a risk of 1 in 5 million of becoming contaminated with AIDS; would you worry about it? Half the respondents indicated that it would worry them. When asked if they would be prepared to make a financial contribution to exclude this risk, almost half (44 percent) said they would be prepared to pay; one-third would be prepared to pay a week's wages or more.

Why does such a minute chance lead people to behave in this way? First, there is a tendency to binary thinking: whether the chance of having something serious is 1 in 100 or 1 in 100,000, a chance is a chance, the argument commonly runs, and even if the chance of a positive result is known to be small, many people will react with "Yes, but suppose that one person is me." Another factor promoting acceptance of this type of technology is that people want to prevent feelings of regret for the choices they make ("I do not want to blame myself later for not having tried everything I could"). This anticipated decision regret gives screening a strongly imperative character.[11]

The social network also plays an important role in people's decisions, which are influenced to a considerable extent by others. In addition, choosing not to use available medical technologies can also have consequences. This was apparent from a study conducted on older pregnant women who consciously decided not to participate in a test for chromosomal abnormalities. Many of the women found it difficult to refuse the technology, a decision they had to defend to the outside world. They realized that nonparticipation could have considerable consequences if they were to give birth to a handicapped child ("It's your own fault").[12]

THE FUTURE OF DUTCH MIDWIFERY

Developments in the medical technological field have strong consequences on the daily routine of Dutch midwives. The technologies enable detection of abnormalities, with new technologies being offered all the time. Scientists and manufacturers cannot wait to have their test methods accepted and applied; pregnant women want to deliver healthy babies, leading them to use the new diagnostic techniques; the government attempts to restrict their use but cannot prevent the diffusion of technology. Moreover, such developments are taking place at a time when liberal ideology is dominant, a time when independence, autonomy, and the right to be informed are central issues: People should be able to choose for themselves which test they wish to undergo.

Medical-technological developments form a strong threat to the Dutch midwifery system, which always placed the natural character of pregnancy at the fore. This leads many midwives to be against the ever-increasing medical-technological interference with pregnant women. Nevertheless, there are a few midwives who favor technology: they are conscious that being able to use it can increase the status and prestige of their occupation. It is striking that some man-midwives are among those who strongly advocate the use of technology.

Science will continue developing and offering choice-giving technologies that may lead to the rise of the "tentative pregnancy."[13] In the future, a woman will not feel or call herself pregnant until the eighteenth week of pregnancy, after all the prenatal tests show favorable results. Will this also happen in the Netherlands, or will the Dutch preoccupation with natural pregnancy lead to a situation in which more and more pregnant women will turn away from the technology? That is for the future to show.

NOTES

1. de Reu, P.A.O.M., "Routinematige toepassing van de echoscopie in de fysiologisch zwangerschap" ("Routine use of ultrasound during normal pregnancy"), *Tijdschrift voor Verloskundigen*, 12 (January 1987): 10–15.
2. Ezinga, G., and D. E. Ezinga-Schotten, "Verloskundigen en de echoscopie" ("Midwives and ultrasound"), *Tijdschrift voor Verloskundigen*, 8 (May 1983): 170–174.
3. Timmermans, A.J.Th., "Routinematig gebruik van scanning in de huispraktijk" ("Routine scanning in normal practice"), *Tijdschrift voor Verloskundigen*, 12 (January 1987): 15–17.
4. Cuppen, A., "Goede verloskunde zonder routine echoscopie" ("Good obstetrics without routine ultrasound"), *Tijdschrift voor Verloskundigen*, 12 (January 1987): 18–24.
5. Exalto, N., and J. W. Wladimiroff, "Routine-echoscopie in de verloskunde?" ("Routine ultrasound in obstetrics?"), *Nederlands Tijdschrift voor Geneeskunde*, 133 (1989): 1439–1441.
6. Kloosterman, M. D., "Prenatale diagnostiek, enige cijfers over de laatste jaren" ("Prenatal diagnosis, some recent data"), *Nederlands Tijdschrift voor Obstetrie en Gynaecologie*, 103 (August 1990): 238–240.
7. Thomassen-Brepols, L. J., *Psychosociale Aspecten van Prenatale Diagnostiek* (*Psychosocial Aspects of Prenatal Diagnosis*), Rotterdam: doctoral dissertation, 1985.
8. Wald, N. J., H. S. Cuckle and J. W. Densem et al, "Maternal serum screening for Down's syndrome in early pregnancy," *British Medical Journal*, 297 (1988): 883–887.
9. Roelofsen, E.C.C., L. I. Kamerbeek and Tj. Tymstra, "Chances and choices. Psycho-social consequences of maternal serum screening. A report from the Netherlands," *Journal of Reproductive and Infant Psychology*, 11 (1993): 41–47.
10. Tymstra, Tj., C. Bajema, J. R. Beekhuis, and A. Mantingh, "Women's opinions on the offer and use of prenatal diagnosis," *Prenatal Diagnosis*, 11 (1991): 893–898.
11. Tymstra, Tj., "The imperative character of medical technology and the meaning of anticipated decision regret", *International Journal of Technology Assessment in Health Care*, 5 (1991): 207–213.
12. Keppels, M., A. S. van der Velde, Tj. Tymstra, and A. Mantingh, "Vlokkentest of vruchtwaterpunctie? Een onderzoek naar het keuzegedrag en de ervaringen van zwangeren" ("Chorionic villi sampling or amniocentesis? An investigation into the decision behavior and experience of expectant mothers"), *Medisch Contact*, 42 (1987): 462–464.
13. Katz Rothman, B., *The Tentative Pregnancy. Prenatal Diagnosis and the Future of Motherhood.* (New York: Viking, 1986).

III

MIDWIVES, MATERNITY
HOME-CARE ASSISTANTS, AND
THE ROLE OF THE STATE

8

Dutch Midwifery, Past and Present: An Overview

Eva Abraham-Van der Mark

Dutch midwives operate as autonomous medical practitioners and have a high professional status. They are, together with general practitioners, responsible for all normal home and clinical deliveries, including prenatal care and caring for mother and child during the lying-in period. Since the seventeenth century, their profession evolved differently from the way it developed in the other European countries and the United States. Although midwives lost ground in the twentieth century in other Western countries, Dutch midwifery was characterized by growing professionalization: midwives' qualifications were increased, standards for recruitment and training were made more rigorous, and their organization gained in power. At the same time, the tradition of working with "low" medical technology was maintained.

HISTORICAL BACKGROUNDS

Early Secularization and the Division of Labor

During the Middle Ages, one of the midwife's main tasks was baptism: to save the soul of the newborn infant who was vulnerable and often succumbed to death in its first hours. The midwife was an instrument of the Church, responsible for the control and discipline of the flock, recruited and supervised by the parish priest and the bishop. Wolfgang Gubalke[1] called his chapter on midwifery during the Middle Ages *Hilfe su Seeligkeit* (Help to Salvation). Writing about France, both Mireille Laget[2] and Jacques Gélis[3] mention "the

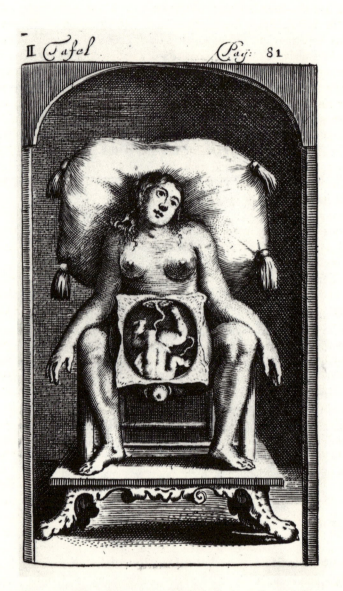

Woman in labor sitting in birthing chair, from Samuel Jans-
sonius, *Korte en Bondige Verhandeling van de Voortteeling
en't Kinderbaren* (*Short and Graphic Description of Labor
and Childbirth*), Amsterdam, 1680.

obsession with baptism," not to let a soul be eternally condemned because its owner had not been baptized. Midwives' sacred and moral tasks did not end with the Middle Ages. During the Counter-Reformation, in Roman Catholic regions, especially in France, supervision by the Church was even more stringent, since midwives were responsible for the detection of any signs of heresy or immorality. In seventeenth-century England, they were deployed in the struggle against various magical practices surrounding pregnancy and birth. In the same century in France, while obstetrics was developed by doctors in the cities that provided a model for other European countries, midwifery in the countryside remained under the control of priests. Heinz Schilling quotes from regulations in a French village (Sarlat in the Dordogne) in 1729, where midwives were recruited and appointed by the priest and had to be "free of any suspicion of heresy, black magic, superstition or any other faults and should have exemplary life style and morals."[4]

During the Dutch Republic (1579–1795),[5] midwives were relieved of the religious duties they had performed since the Middle Ages and were established as a medical occupation. With Calvinism as the dominant religion, midwives were no longer even allowed to perform the important rite of baptism. This rite had to take place in the Church, within the religious community, and could not be performed by women. This was indeed a radical change, which initially met with a great deal of resistance in the Calvinists' own circles.

One of the main characteristics of the Dutch Republic was the separation between State and Church. The State was now expected to be exclusively concerned with its citizens' well-being on Earth, whereas the care of their souls resided under the Church. All legislation and jurisdiction became the direct concern of the State, although in fact they were delegated to the local authorities. With the regulation of medicine a municipal responsibility, various towns appointed physicians whose duty it was to control medical practice, including midwifery. Midwives working in towns (Delft, Amsterdam, Leiden, and others) were regulated by town councils that laid down ordinances and fees to be paid per delivery (Marland in this volume). In 1668, Amsterdam made the midwives' examination by the *Collegium Obstetricum* compulsory. Midwives' tasks were medical and hygienic, and they were no longer responsible to priests but to doctors appointed by the town council. Instead of being allies of priests, midwives became allies of doctors. The criteria for recruitment were no longer piety but citizenship, marital status (married or widowed), a good reputation, and knowledge of reading and writing plus practical experience in attending deliveries.[6]

Schilling states that the early secularization of midwives' tasks meant a radical break with the Middle Ages and the beginning of a process of profound change in mentality. He argues that it heralded an important step towards professionalization and made midwifery in the Dutch Republic an example for other countries. Especially in moments of crisis, it must have been crucial that the midwife was to concentrate on the mother rather than worrying about saving the soul of the unborn infant.

In the eighteenth century, obstetrics was no longer the exclusive domain of women, since men began to assist delivering babies. In Germany and France, as well as in England, a new type of surgeon appeared, the master of obstetrics, man-midwife, or accoucheur. This profession was also introduced in the Netherlands. Usually the masters of obstetrics or man-midwives performed the more complicated deliveries. They had more qualifications than women, were authorized to use instruments (such as various hooks and screws, and in some cases, early predecessors of the forceps), and had the right to ask higher fees. They also gave instruction to midwives.[7]

In the Netherlands, the general division of labor was for *medicinae doctores* to be advisers in obstetric problems; midwives could make use of this advice if they were able to apply it without the use of instruments, which was explicitly prohibited to them. If it was decided that in a particular case instruments had to be used, the man-midwife was the one to do so. M. J. Van Lieburg and Hilary Marland[11] point out that in the eighteenth century, the occupational boundaries of midwives and man-midwives were clearly demarcated: "What characterizes these professions is permission (or its absence) to use certain obstetric instruments. Except for the enema syringe and the catheter, midwives were not allowed to use any instruments."[8] In reality, the application of these rules and regulations differed from town to town and region to region. The famous midwife, Catharina Schrader, who practiced from 1693 to 1745, used the instruments that her deceased husband, a surgeon, had left her (various hooks for taking out an infant that had died in the uterus).[9] However, because the prohibition against using instruments remained the standard, midwives appear to have specialized in manual techniques to deal with complicated deliveries. Schrader's diary makes it clear that, although she worked closely together with surgeons and doctors, she knew how to deal with various malrepresentations. Through "the art" of manipulation, she successfully managed various breech deliveries, as well as deliveries of twins and in one case triplets.[10]

Other eighteenth-century midwives who wrote about their experiences, Willemina Waltman of Dordrecht[11] and Elisabeth and Neeltje van Putten of Rotterdam,[12] also appear to have had considerable manual capabilities. Waltman dealt successfully with various face, breech, foot, and knee presentations. Her list of thirty-six babies presented in a transverse position includes arm, stomach, and one back presentation. Of the fifty-three twins delivered by Waltman, twenty-nine presented abnormally. Elisabeth and Neeltje van Putten, daughters of a prominent surgeon, were exceptional because they graduated not only as midwives, but also obtained permission to exercise the obstetric practice of the man-midwife.[13] Neeltje, moreover, published two articles in the Dutch medical periodical *Hippocrates*, established by three doctors.[14] The periodical was dedicated to fighting the increased use of instruments. Although Neeltje herself was entitled to apply the forceps, she pleaded for a sparing use of this tool and emphasized that most often it is best to be patient and trust that eventually nature will take its course, even in difficult births: "Even if the forceps works in a single case, how many are the cases where it does not, and how many women and infants died from its use? It is far better to allow Nature to take its course."[15]

In *Hippocrates*, editor Jacobus Johannes Walop criticized the advance of medical technology of the period.[16] His article, "Remarks about the Simplification of Obstetrics," is against the inappropriate and common use of instruments. It ends by stating that many problems could have been avoided by leaving childbirth in the hands of women. They are the ones who are most suited to guide the birth process and possess the necessary "patience and gentleness—the talents for being able to wait" that make them better birth attendants than men.[17] Walop also stated that well-trained midwives should be allowed to apply obstetric manual techniques, such as version and extraction. In brief, Walop advocated restricting the use of technology in obstetrics in favor of births without artificial aids. Van Lieburg and Marland point out that other masters in obstetrics, such as Matthias van Geuns (1735–1817), Jacob Denijs (1681–1741), and his student Cornelius Terne (1778–93) (master in obstetrics and *doctor medicinae* at Leiden), also advocated improving the position of the midwife by establishing a thorough course of instruction and promulgating "natural" childbirth. Various authors (Schilling, Van Lieburg, Gerrit-Jan Kloosterman,[18] and Helena Van der Borg) suggest that in the seventeenth and eighteenth centuries in the Netherlands, although rivalry between men and women in obstetrics existed and the power balance was very uneven, the relationship between them was characterized by cooperation and consciousness of mutual dependency to a greater extent than in other European countries.

The Nineteenth Century, Low Social Status and High Level of Autonomy

(*For a more detailed discussion of midwifery and obstetrics in the nineteenth century, read the chapters by Marland and Anja Hiddinga.*)

Midwives were regulated by the Laws of 1818 and 1865 (*see* Marland in this volume). The prohibition on the use of instruments was reiterated, and the Law of 1865 restated a clause of the Act of 1818, that "midwives are only to attend such deliveries that are the work of nature or which can be executed by hand. They may not use any instruments." Another article of the law added: "Nor shall they prescribe, advise, or offer any internal or external medicines, nor perform any bloodletting." Only setting enemas and using the catheter were permitted to the midwife.[19]

Van Lieburg and Marland[20] conclude that in the nineteenth century, midwifery and obstetrics in the Netherlands incorporated a number of features that set them apart from other European countries and the United States: "Perhaps the most striking divergences were the early introduction of legislation control and licensing for both male and female obstetric practitioners, the institutionalization of midwife training, and the very low incidence of hospital births."[21] Although the majority of all women gave birth at home, in Germany, France, and England, clinics for the poor (*maternités*, or lying-in clinics) were growing in numbers. This development did not occur in the Netherlands (Lumey in this volume). The clinical schools in Amsterdam and Rotterdam were very unpopular because of high maternal and infant mortality.[22] Moreover, these institutions were considered as not consonant with Dutch national character.[23]

In the Law of 1865, the midwife was declared indispensable. Legal regulation came early and without much commotion. It meant, however, an end to any exceptions to the rule that prohibited midwives' involvement in complicated deliveries. Moreover, after 1865, midwives came increasingly under the control and authority of male medical practitioners.[24] J. J. Klinkert points out that, faced with increasing competition with doctors, midwives lacked the assertiveness and organization to defend their professional interests.[25] They came largely from the lower middle class. Twenty percent of them had been domestic servants. The majority were daughters of farmers, shopkeepers, and laborers and, unlike nursing, the profession did not attract any women of the upper classes.[26] It appears that although some upper-middle-class and upper-class women entered nursing, they did not become midwives, perhaps because of the low status of the profession, the irregular hours, and the autonomy or "freedom" of the midwife to go out on her own at any hour of the day or night in lower-class neighborhoods. This freedom was held against her. For women of the bourgeoisie, walking in the streets without male protection was considered inappropriate.[27] Nursing and midwifery developed separately and have remained distinct up to the present.

Midwives' lives were not easy because they worked long hours for meager salaries and were held in low regard. Yet they retained a high level of autonomy, and the establishment of midwife colleges ensured good training (Marland in this volume). In the nineteenth century, the midwives' position was consolidated, firmly anchored within the Dutch system of obstetric care.

THE TWENTIETH CENTURY

The Monopoly of 1941

It was in the twentieth century that Dutch obstetrics and midwifery became most distinct from other Western industrialized countries. Alarmed by the steady increase in the percentages of home deliveries managed by general practitioners (with higher costs), legislation was drafted in 1925 to protect midwives against the competition of doctors. However, in 1953 Muntendam,

Secretary of Health, emphasized that the argument in favor of the midwives' monopoly was not based on cost, but rather the higher quality of the obstetric care they provide. He stated that midwives were better trained in obstetrics than general practitioners and that they had the right professional attitude: "They can assist at birth with patience—still the most important condition for normal obstetrics."[28] During the German occupation of the Netherlands, the *Ziekenfondsen* (the Dutch national health insurance system that covers 65 percent of the population) was established. The board of this institution decided in 1941 to give midwives a monopoly over normal obstetrics, without the use of instruments. This marked an important advance in midwives' position. The monopoly implies that in normal home deliveries the insurance pays for the services of a midwife, which includes all prenatal and postnatal care. A general practitioner may be called in if no midwife is available in the municipality. Hospitalization is only covered where there is some evidence or suspicion of a problem. Women who have private insurance are free to choose between delivery at home or in a hospital, and between the services of a midwife and a general practitioner. Since the early 1980s, however, the national health insurance system (*Ziekenfondsen*) reimburses women who prefer the short-stay hospital delivery to home birth, thus giving them greater freedom of choice.

Because the Dutch system of national health insurance was set up during the occupation of the Netherlands in World War II, protest against the decision of the *Ziekenfondsen* was not possible at that time. In 1947, however, the issue of the midwives' monopoly came up for confirmation by the Ministry of Health. Among the points raised in the preceding debate were: midwives' qualifications, the right of all women, whatever their means, to be free to choose between the services of a midwife and a general practitioner, and the role of the State in protecting one particular professional group.

The outcome was that the midwives kept their monopoly. A compromise giving the pregnant woman a fixed sum of money and the choice of spending it on either a midwife or a general practitioner (in the latter case supplementing the difference in cost from her own means) was rejected. The decision made by the *Ziekenfondsen*, often referred to as the "German Law," was maintained but did not actually become a law until 1966.

Klinkert has pointed out that when the Health Law of 1865 was passed, the position of midwives had been decided upon without consulting them.[29] In 1947, however, the midwives had two organizations: the Roman Catholic Association of Midwives, founded in 1921, and the Union of Dutch Midwives of 1926. Through their unions, they were better able to defend their interests. In 1947, the special number of the *Journal of Practical Midwifery (Maandblad voor Praktische Verloskunde)*,[30] which was dedicated to the debate on the decree of 1941, opened with a short statement from the journal's editors announcing that the midwives were ready to fight for their rights. However, in the letter that followed, which was signed by the secretaries of the two unions, the midwives appeared rather hesitant, pointing out the great amount of support they received from obstetricians, and claiming that the real issue was not professional interest but the well-being of the Dutch population. The remainder of the journal was filled with letters from the directors of the midwife schools and other obstetricians offering staunch support to the midwives' cause by pointing to their expertise in normal obstetrics. It was emphasized that compared to general practitioners midwives spend more time on each delivery and that deliveries managed by general practitioners showed higher percentages of intervention. There was only one letter, "A deviant voice," that defended the interests of the general practitioners.[31] The midwives' monopoly of 1941 proved to be firm protection during the difficult 1960s and 1970s, when the medicalization of obstetric care became manifest.

Midwives, General Practitioners, and Obstetricians

In the 1950s, the high birth rates muted conflicts between midwives and doctors, although competition between them did exist, particularly in rural areas. Since the early 1960s, however, the birth rate dropped dramatically, and the number of midwives, obstetricians, and general practitioners started to rise. Between 1972 and 1982, the number of midwives increased 12 percent, general practitioners 22, and obstetricians 64.[32] This has resulted in considerable changes in the division of labor among the three groups. A larger percentage of births are now attended by obstetricians and take place in hospitals. The percentage of deliveries done by midwives has increased somewhat, whereas the general practitioners have lost ground.

	Obstetrical assistance (percentages)		
	General Practitioner	*Midwife*	*Obstetrician*
1960	46.9	37.2	16.7
1970	34.9	36.7	27.8
1975	23.0	39.7	37.3
1980	15.7	40.6	41.0
1989	14	43	43
1991	11	44	45

(Hessing-Wagner, J. C., *Samenhang in de zorg rond geboorte en jonge kinderen*, and by the same author, *Geboorte en zorgvernieuwing* (Rijswijk: Sociaal en Cultureel Planbureau, 1985 and 1991).

In the 1960s and 1970s, relations among the three professional groups became highly competitive, and the midwives' monopoly was attacked by general practitioners. With increasing unemployment among them, some general practitioners tried to reclaim tasks and reconquer territory. They demanded that their tasks in prenatal and postnatal care should be increased, and one of them even stated that not attending deliveries contributed to an identity crisis.[33] In 1972, however, a report entitled "Recommendations for Obstetric Care," written at the request of the Ministry of Health, confirmed that midwives were more expert at normal obstetrics than general practitioners. Moreover, it was stated that, with the decreased number of births and the increased number of medical students, it would not be possible to improve the students' training in obstetrics. Because of inadequate training and lack of experience in delivering babies in their practice, general practitioners had undergone a deprofessionalization process in this field, and many had decided to stop attending deliveries altogether. J. I. de Neeff stated as early as 1973 in his doctoral dissertation: "It is irresponsible for the majority of the general practitioners to attend deliveries along with their many other pressing duties. They should leave this to the midwives."[34] In the 1990s, general practitioners are divided on the issue of attending deliveries. Most of them have given up obstetric care, although a minority wants to reclaim obstetric tasks. The number of general practitioners who attend deliveries decreases annually, especially in the cities.

Prenatal care is the domain of the midwife. She is trained to do the standard examinations and is proficient in recognizing potential abnormalities. During prenatal care, it is decided which women can safely give birth at home. In making this decision, midwives and obstetricians are not always in agreement. Competition between them is concentrated in the blurring of boundaries between normal and pathological. The list of medical indications named after G. J. Kloosterman provided guidelines to screen for hospitalization (Treffers in this volume), and for the division of labor between midwives and general practitioners (who take care of normal or physiological deliveries) and obstetricians (who attend those showing pathology). The revision of the list (1987) recognizes three categories of pregnancy: low-, medium-, and high-risk. Women with low-risk pregnancies can give birth at home, which has proven to be the best protection against medical intervention. Women with high-risk pregnancies, on the other hand, are referred to a fully equipped obstetric department. Medium-risk women are sent to an obstetrician for one consultation. Depending on its outcome, the midwife decides whether she will keep the woman under her care or refer her to the obstetrician.[35]

Since the revision of 1987, the midwife has gained a considerable amount of decision-making power. She is now formally entitled to define what is normal and abnormal (before 1987, this was the obstetrician's privilege), and she is the one who makes the final decision. Although midwives in the cities do not view this as changing their relationship with obstetricians, the revision is a formal confirmation of what was the status quo for many, if not all midwives. Therefore, it is an important step towards becoming a full profession, that is, having control over one's work.[36] The revision of the list of medical indications in 1987 caused considerable commotion and resulted in an official protest by the professional obstetric organization, but the decision made by the *Raad van Ziekenfondsen* (board of the national health insurance) in favor of the midwives was maintained.[37] In the 1980s, the State has consistently supported the midwives' position, partly but not exclusively because their lower costs were attractive in a period of severe cuts in spending on health care.

Recruitment and Training

An important strategy in the midwives' professionalization is their education, which aims at enabling the midwife to function autonomously. The criteria for recruitment as well as the curriculum have repeatedly been made more rigorous.

There are three colleges for midwives, in Amsterdam, Rotterdam, and Heerlen, in the southern part of the country. It is difficult to be admitted to any of them. Each year, the number of applicants exceeds by far the number of available places. Annually, the three institutions select an average of seventy-five new students from approximately 1,000 applicants. These must have at least five years of secondary education with A grades in chemistry and biology. Moreover, through interviews, applicants are screened for personal characteristics.[38] About 80 percent of all students obtain the license and take the Hippocratic oath, which leads to independent practice. Men were only admitted to midwifery colleges in the 1970s, and by 1991, the ratio of men who practiced midwifery was still low: thirty-six compared to 1,115 women.[39]

Today the training course lasts three years, with theoretical and practical work combined each year. Theory includes chemistry, anatomy, human physiology, obstetrics, pediatrics, gynecology, family planning, psychology, and sociology. Training is planned to take four years in 1993. Each school is allied to a large obstetrical and gynecological unit that specializes in low- and high-risk pregnancies and deliveries. Students receive practical training in these units, as well as with midwives who have a private practice. They are required to perform forty supervised deliveries before they can take the licensing examination.[40]

From the beginning of midwife schools, the directors have been male obstetricians. This changed when a female obstetrician was appointed in Amsterdam in the 1970s. After her retirement in 1991, she was replaced by a midwife, and it was decided that in the future, only midwives will be eligible to apply for a vacancy in the directorship at one of the three schools. This control over training is another advance in the midwives' professionalization. One of them commented: "We are no longer led by the obstetricians, now it is time to be on our own."

The midwives' training course is completely separate from nursing. These occupations evolved separately, and there is an essential difference in orientation and outlook. Kloosterman said at the fiftieth anniversary of the International Association of Midwives: "The obedient female assistant who needs the doctor's presence at the end of a normal childbirth in a healthy woman can be called a nurse or a nurse-midwife. But a midwife she is not, no more than the experienced surgical nurse is a surgeon." A midwife stated:

> The professions of nursing and midwifery are direct opposites. While one is devoted to care for the sick, injured, and dying within a hospital, the other assumes care of the normal, healthy woman and her infant at home. The midwife and the nurse-midwife come to a birth with different points of view. The midwife has chosen her job because she prefers to work with healthy mothers as an independent practitioner. By the very nature of her job she is unsuited to take orders unquestioningly.

Midwives' Work

In the twentieth century, midwives' qualifications have been increased at various times. In 1991, midwives attended 45 percent of all deliveries. They are required to give prenatal care, care during labor and delivery, and postnatal care independently of other health-care professionals. Only if complications arise is the woman or baby referred to an obstetrician or pediatrician. Midwives attend deliveries independently at home and in hospitals. Those working in private practice come to the hospital to attend clients during labor and delivery. Moreover, 15 percent of all midwives are hospital employed.

The midwife's task is directed towards the prevention of unnecessary medical intervention and, wherever possible, the prevention of pathology. Midwives are expected to function as psychological and social counselors for their clients, and must be reluctant to intervene in the birth process. They emphasize the importance of their psychological and social tasks, such as boosting the self-confidence of the mother and creating a tranquil atmosphere, and state that it is essential for the woman in labor to feel that she is in control in order to give birth effectively and without fear. It is assumed that this will prevent a considerable amount of pathology.

The method used by midwives is known as the physiological approach,[41] and is based on the principle that in human beings, pregnancy and birth are essentially normal physiological processes that generally require only good prenatal care and counseling. Continuity of care is considered essential: ideally, a woman sees the same midwife during her entire pregnancy, labor, delivery, and lying-in period. With the increasing number of group practices, this becomes more difficult.[42] Midwife Astrid Limburg, however, states that in her practice in Amsterdam: "The pregnant woman and her partner visit the three of us to establish a bond of confidence and avoid feelings of disappointment if one of us is absent."

On the basis of her observations of prenatal care in Mexico, the United States, Sweden, and Holland, Brigitte Jordan comments:

> What is striking about prenatal consultations with midwives is that, in general, they are conducted in an atmosphere that is much more relaxed, unhurried, supportive, and personal than is usually the case in medical consultations. Part of this effect may come simply from the greater openness of woman-to-woman interaction; another reason may be reduction of the social distance between lay patient and professional physician. Though many midwives, through training and long experience, know more about normal pregnancy and birth than many a doctor, their lower professional status avoids many of the problems inherent in the conventional patient-doctor relationship.[43]

In 1990, 15 percent of all midwives were employed by hospitals, whereas 71 percent were established in independent practice. Of the latter, 37 percent had a solo practice; the others worked as partners or in a group practice. The group practices are increasing the fastest.[44] The midwife must be available at any hour, day or night, through a physician's or messaging service. What is attractive about a group practice is that the required twenty-four-hour availability and readiness can be divided among several colleagues. Fourteen percent of midwives work as permanent substitutes in an established practice. Hospital employment has been severely criticized among midwives themselves, but its more regular working hours appear to offer a way out for those who are married, especially those who have young children.[45]

Midwives are socialized to view their work as a vocation rather than an occupation. However, the ideal of total dedication and continuous availability is in conflict with the desire for better working conditions and a private life. Sixty percent of all midwives are younger than forty,[46] which indicates a high dropout rate. The profession is difficult to combine with a family of one's own. Moreover, various unmarried midwives in their late thirties and early forties register at universities to start new careers. The Dutch Organization of Midwives (NOV) plans to carry out a survey to explore these issues, because it fears that the present shortage of midwives may endanger the system of home birth. The organization aims at lessening the average work load of 165 deliveries a year to 127. Midwives' work is extremely demanding, and the financial rewards are far from satisfying.[47]

Medical Technology

Although there is an increase in the professionalization of midwives, their use of technology has remained extremely limited. For prenatal care, their technology includes a wooden "trumpet" (monoauricular stethoscope) for listening to fetal heart sounds, the doptone (which registers fetal heart sounds by means of sound waves, and can be used much earlier in pregnancy than the "trumpet"), a sphygmometer, stethoscope, blood-taking equipment (the blood is tested in a laboratory), strips for testing urine, and a scale. The kit that the midwife takes with her to a woman in labor consists of two *kochers* (which ideally are used only for cutting the umbilical cord), needles and suturing equipment in case an episiotomy is required, resuscitation equipment and oxygen, sterile gloves, a scale to weigh the baby, and a few medicines.[48] The mother is given a list of articles that she must have ready for the birth. These are simple, cheap objects that can serve various purposes and are available to everyone.[49]

Midwives who prefer an upright position for births advocate the birth stool as "new" technology, even though its early predecessors appeared on woodcuts as early as the Middle Ages. In the 1980s, modern versions of this stool have been developed. At an international obstetric congress in 1989 in Amsterdam, a simple plastic birthing stool was displayed alongside the latest gynecological chair.

Whenever anyone asks a midwife about the instruments she uses, she will often hold her hands up: "You must measure the uterus with your hands, which will help you to feel how big the child is and what its position is. No instrument can replace your hands." "Being able to depend on your hands, that is the most important" is a frequent remark. Thus, midwifery is described as a craft of "feeling"—a manual art.

Since the nineteenth century, however, seeing has become increasingly more important in medicine. In 1880, the English doctor Meadows stated: "Seeing is believing and, in a realistic age like the present, it might also be said that not seeing is not believing." This trend continued, and it is not only the uterus that is no longer terra incognita, but also the fetus within has become visible. In the course of the 1980s, seeing has become part of the usual method of prenatal care. Dutch midwives are divided about ultrasound technology, however,[50] and the board of their professional organization has not voiced an opinion in this regard.[51]

In the last decade, several articles and letters appeared in the midwives' professional journal on the subject of ultrasound, and in 1988, the Dutch Organization for Midwives held a seminar in which advocates and opposition were given an opportunity to speak. Many of the comments became highly emotional. Is it chance that the one who is strongly dedicated to propagating this technology is a man-midwife? He gave added weight to his comments at the seminar by saying that midwives have to go with the times.[52] Some of those opposed to the routine use of ultrasound explained that even though an advertising slogan for ultrasound machines says "happiness is in a small box," the technology can change pregnancy into a time of tension and insecurity. Ultrasound is intended to diagnose phenomena that are not amenable to therapy; if there are really problems, abortion is the only solution.[53] Ultrasound can, however, cause worry even in less severe instances. One midwife, W. J. Meijer, quoted the following couple: "We don't understand anything about the ultrasound tests; first the child is growing and then it has shrunk. How is that possible? But it does make you very worried and uneasy. You wonder whether the child will be all right."[54]

A. Cuppen, another midwife, concluded that it would be better for midwives to improve the human aspects of midwifery than to concentrate on technology.[55] She encouraged an emphasis on the psycho-social approach directed towards the autonomy of the woman during labor, the bonding of mother and child, and encouraging the father to play an active role during childbirth. Meijer closed her testimony by saying:

> What must we midwives do now? Should we join the group of intra-uterine tourists or engineers who wish to take complete advantage of all technology that appears on the market? Or should we keep the wisdom of the midwife within our profession by using intervention only when we absolutely must? Only then will expectant mothers be reassured, and only thus will we keep physiological obstetrics in the *safe* and *experienced hands of the midwife*. Are our hands not the most beautiful and the most precious instruments that we own?[56]

Organization

The Dutch Organization of Midwives was founded in 1975, and is the result of a fusion between the Roman Catholic Association of Midwives and the Union of Dutch Midwives. The organization is an advocate for midwives' interests and aims at improving the quality of normal obstetric care. In the last two decades, it has become more powerful, fighting effectively for full professionalization.[57] Participation on the local and national levels has increased considerably. One group of assertive young midwives licensed in 1978, seriously concerned about the rapid increase in the percentage of deliveries in hospitals, started "Working Group 78." Through campaigns in the media, lectures at home and abroad (especially the United States and Canada), the publication of brochures and books, and even documentary films, they publicized the importance of home birth and its emotional advantages to women. These midwives drew large audiences at international conferences. They maintain a "Foreign Office" in Amsterdam that distributes information all over the world. It also briefs visitors from abroad on the system of home birth, and invites them to accompany a practicing midwife during prenatal care and deliveries.

CONCLUSION

It has often been stated that the invention of the forceps in the seventeenth century marked the beginning of the decline of midwifery. Midwives were excluded from its use (even though there have always been exceptions to this rule) as well as from other obstetric instruments, which only men, surgeons, and doctors were allowed to apply. Although the use value of the early forceps must have been ineffectual,[58] they had great symbolic value and were an important source of power and prestige. The emergence of prestigious techniques and methods goes together with a technical and social differentiation between those who can avail themselves of these techniques and those who cannot. In obstetrics, this also implied a differentiation between men and women. Although Dutch midwives were prohibited from using instruments, the emphasis was that for normal births, these were unnecessary, undesirable, and dangerous. All ordinances, decrees, and laws distinguish between normal births (the midwife's sphere of action) and complicated, pathological births (the doctor's field). This distinction between physiology and pathology is the basis of the present Dutch obstetric system (Treffers in this volume) and its accommodation of low technology (employed by the midwife) and high technology (used by obstetricians).

In the twentieth century, with increasing medicalization, midwives in most Western countries lost ground and obstetrics became dominated by doctors employing high technology. Dutch midwives, on the contrary, have reached full professional status, and Dutch obstetricians are divided among themselves: Although many of them are in favor of further hospitalization, the majority support home birth attended by a midwife. The divisions within occupational groups (general practitioners as well as obstetricians) show that the Anglo-Saxon conflict models that have been used to describe the relations between midwives and doctors should not be applied to Dutch obstetrics. Barbara Katz Rothman, for example, described midwifery and medicine in the United States as antagonistic, impossible to combine and reconcile.[59] This does not hold true for the Dutch situation, which is characterized by recurring conflicts about occupational boundaries but has never known efforts to abolish the midwife or squeeze her out of independent practice (*see* also Marland in this volume).

Ideology (the belief in science, progress, conquering nature) is the driving force behind the success of high medical technology.[60] In the Netherlands, however, this ideology was countered by the view of pregnancy and birth as normal physiological processes.

Since the 1970s, Dutch midwives have gained in popularity. Consistent support from the State and from various obstetricians, advanced professionalization, and a powerful organization have contributed to their present position as an independent medical profession. Also important are the increased assertiveness of health consumers, the increased criticism of medical practitioners by the women's movement, and criticism of the medicalization of birth and praise for Dutch midwives in many countries. Dutch midwives receive favorable attention from the World Health Organization,[61] because they provide high-quality prenatal and postnatal care and strive for continuity of care, they emphasize the essential criterion of a good personal relationship between mother and midwife, they reject routine preparations (enema, bath, shave) for labor, they encourage alternative birth positions (such as the upright position if the mother prefers it), and they stand for a low intervention rate.

Some authors,[62] and the midwives themselves at various points in history, have interpreted the prohibition on using instruments as a disadvantage and as discrimination. Since the 1980s, however, midwives and the majority of doctors emphasize the advantages of physiological obstetrics, which is antipathetic to instruments and medication for normal births. Midwives aim at assisting healthy women to give birth autonomously and to protect them against any unnecessary intervention. The use of instruments would make their practice implausible, and lead to increased medicalization and to intense competition with obstetricians. With growing skepticism and discontent about the medicalization of pregnancy and birth, midwives' low-tech approach appears to be an important resource of power.

NOTES

1. Gubalke, Wolfgang, *Die Hebamme in Wandel der Zeiten* (Hannover: Staude, 1964).

2. Laget, Mireille, *Naissance, l'accouchement avant l'age de la clinique* (Paris: Editions du Seuil, 1982).

3. Gélis, Jacques, *L'arbre et le fruit: la naissance dans l'Occident moderne (XVIe–XIXe siècle)* (Paris: Fayard, 1984).

4. Schilling, Heinz, *"Religion und Gesellschaft in der Calvinistischen Republik der Vereinigten Niederlande,"* in *Kirche und Gesellschaftlicher Wandel in Deutschen und Niederländischen Stadten der Neuzeit,* Petri, Franz (ed.) (Cologne, Vienna: Bohlau Verlag, 1980): 197–250.

5. The Dutch Republic was the outcome of a struggle for independence from the rule of the Habsburg family, whose reign extended as far as Spain and the Spanish-American colonies. The Republic ended in 1795 and was followed by a period of French domination. The Dutch state became a monarchy in 1815.

6. Van Lieburg, M. J., and Hilary Marland, "Midwife regulation, education, and the practice in the Netherlands during the nineteenth century," *Medical History,* 33 (1989 A): 296–317; Marland, Hilary, "The midwife in the town and countryside in eighteenth-century Holland," in Marland, Hilary (ed.), *The Art of Midwifery: Early Modern Midwives in Europe and North America* (London/New York: Routledge, 1993).

7. Van der Borg, 1992; Van Lieburg, M. J., "Het Verloskundig onderwijs te Rotterdam voor 1828," in Scholte, E., M. J. van Lieburg, and R. O. Aalbersberg (eds.), *Rijkskweekschool voor vroedvrouwen te Rotterdam, 1882–1982* (Leidschendam: Ministerie van Volksgezondheid en Milieuhygiene, 1982): 5–20; Hilary Marland, 1993.

8. Van Lieburg, M. J., and Hilary Marland, "Elisabeth en Neeltje van Putten: Twee 18e-Eeuwse grensgangers tussen de beroepsvelden van vroedvrouw en vroedmeester," *Tijdschrift voor de Geschiedenis der Geneeskunde, Natuurwetenschappen, Wiskunde en Techniek,* 12 (4), (1989 B): 181–197, quotation 184–185.

9. Van Lieburg, M. J., C. G. Schraders' Memoryboeck van de Vrouwens, Het noti- tieboek van een Friese Vroedvrouw, 1693–1745 (Amsterdam: Rodopi, 1984).

10. See also Schama, Simon, "Making babies safe(ly): The Diary of a Dutch Mid- wife," in The Embarrassment of Riches, chapter 7, iv (New York: Fontana Press, 1987): 517–544.

11. Van Lieburg and Marland, (1989 A): 303–304.

12. Ibid. (1989 B).

13. "The case of the female man-midwives of Rotterdam is of special significance due to the local tradition of trying to reform surgical and obstetrical practice not via the academic branch of medicine but by the surgeons themselves, not from above but from below. Moreover, it offers a remarkable alternative solution to the problem of determining the boundaries between the two areas of obstetric practice." (Van Lieburg and Marland, 1989A): 196–197.

14. Christiaan August Lodewijk Sander (1784–1865), George Hendrik Wachter (1791–1864), and Jacobus Johannes Walop (1788?–1815?), Van Lieburg and Marland, (1989 B): 189.

15. Ibid., p. 191.

16. Ibid., pp. 189–190.

17. Ibid., p. 189.

18. Kloosterman, G. J., "De verloskunde in Vrouw Schrader's 'Memoryboeck,'" in C. G. Schrader's Memoryboeck van de Vrouwens (Amsterdam: Rodopi, 1984): 47–79.

19. In the seventeenth century, the books by foreign midwives, such as Louise Bourget (French) and Justine Sigemundin (German), were translated by Dutch mas- ters of obstetrics directly after their publication. The most prominent among these masters were Cornelis van Solingen (1641–87) and Hendrik van Deventer (1651– 1724). Van Deventer's book Novum Lumen Exhibentes Obstantetricum appeared si- multaneously in Latin and Dutch, and became an international classic. Both these prestigious figures aimed at elevating the midwives through better teaching and training, and promoting the cooperation between them and the masters of obstetrics.

20. Van Lieburg and Marland (1989 A): 305; Klinkert, J. J., Verloskundigen en Artsen, (Alphen a.d.Rijn: Stafleu's Wetenschappelijke Uitgeversmij, 1980): 40.

21. Van Lieburg and Marland (1989 A): 314.

22. Verdoorn, J. A., Het gezondheidswezen te Amsterdam in de 19de Eeuw (Nijmegen: SUN, 1981): 109–112.

23. Sikkel, A., Epiloog, in Scholte, van Lieburg, Aalbersberg, (1982): 200.

24. Van Lieburg and Marland (1989 A): 317.

25. Klinkert, p. 40.

26. Van Lieburg and Marland (1989 A): 316; Van Gelder, Floor, "Is dat nu typies vrouwenwerk? De maatschappelijke positie van vroedvrouwen," Tijdschrift voor Vrou- wenstudies, 3 (1982): 5–33.

27. de Swaan, Abram, De Mens is de Mens een Zorg (Amsterdam: Meulenhoff, 1983): 85–90.

28. Quoted in Crebas, Aya, Beroepskrachtenvoorziening Nota I (Den Bilt: Nederlandse Organisatie van Verloskundigen, 1992): 38.

29. Klinkert, pp. 57–58.

30. Tijdschrift voor Praktische Verloskunde 4 (1947): 97–104.

31. Holmer, A.J.M., "A deviant voice," 1947 *Tijdschrift voor Praktische Verloskunde*, 4, (1947): 103–104; and *Medisch Contact*, 8 (1947): 126–127.

32. Butter, I., and Lapré, R. M., "Verloskundige zorg in Nederland. Vraagverschuiving en Kosten," *Economisch Statistische Berichten* (January 15, 1986): 61–65.

33. Springer, M., "Devaluatie taak huisarts bij verloskundige zorg." *Medisch Contact*, 34 (1980): 1021–1025.

34. de Neeff, J. I., *Prenatale Zorg en het gezondheidscentrum van Didam* (Zevenaar: Uitgeverij Rebers, 1972).

35. A midwife is free to choose an obstetrician (subject to a client's preference) and designate a hospital for a short-stay delivery or for emergency medical care if the need arises. Midwife Astrid Limburg commented:

> We refer clients to all hospitals in town, except one that we consider too medicalized. We work together with about 35 different obstetricians whom we know and respect. We have a good working relationship with them. If there happens to be an obstetrician who we consider too medicalized or who does not give the kind of care that we expect, we make him aware of this. If he does not change, we do not refer clients to him any more. But if a midwife refers a woman too late to an obstetrician, he will criticize her. In this way we correct each other.

Of course, in small communities with fewer midwives and obstetricians, there is more mutual dependence and less freedom to choose between different professionals.

36. Van der Hulst, Leonie, "Het Vroedvrouwenberoep: beroep of professie?" *Tijdschrift voor Verloskundigen* (April 1991): 398–404.

37. Riteco, J. A. and L. Hingstman, *Evaluatie Invoering "Verloskundige Indicatielijst"* (Utrecht: NIVEL, 1991).

38. Crebas, 1992.

39. Hessing-Wagner, J. C., *Geboorte en zorgvernieuwing* (Rijswijk: Sociaal en Cultureel Planbureau, 1991).

40. Information provided by Kweekschool voor Vroedvrouwen, Amsterdam; *see* also Crebas, A., *Beroepsomschrijving Verloskundigen* (Bilthoven: Nederlandse Organisatie van Verloskundigen, 1990).

41. Crebas, A., "De professionele identiteit van de verloskundige," *Tijdschrift voor Verloskundigen*, May and June (1990): 162–200.

42. Dujardin, Rita, *Moederende Verloskundigen, de spanning tussen beroep en gezin* (University of Amsterdam: Vakgroep Sociologie, unpublished manuscript, 1991).

43. Jordan, Brigitte, *Birth in Four Cultures* (Montreal: Eden Press Women's Publications, 1978): 40.

44. Hessing-Wagner, 1991, p. 16.

45. Dujardin, 1991.

46. Hessing-Wagner, 1991, p. 16.

47. The midwife, who theoretically earns about 55,000 guilders (before taxes) per year ($27,500), is expected to work 324 days per year, but most midwives do not earn that much; the true average is about 29,000 guilders (about $14,500), which is a little above the Dutch minimum for single taxpayers. Rita Dujardin note 27, 60–61.

48. Inventory of medical technology in a midwife practice in Amsterdam. For *prenatal care*:

> Wooden "trumpet" (monoauricular or single-ear stethoscope, Pinard) to listen to fetal heart sounds (for use from the twenty-fourth week of pregnancy).

Doptone, to listen to fetal heart sounds by means of sound waves (for use after the twelfth week of pregnancy).

Sphygmometer (to measure blood pressure).

Equipment to take blood samples. (This is done at the first visit. The blood is tested in a laboratory.) At later stages (the twenty-eighth and thirty-sixth weeks of pregnancy), the woman's hemoglobin level is tested.

Paper strips covered with chemicals to test the urine for albumin and glucose.

Scale.

Speculum.

For *labor and birth*:

Monoauricular stethoscope (Pinard).

If upright birth is preferred, a birth stool.

Kit consisting of a "half" *Kocher* (a particular type of scissor) to break the amniotic sac if necessary.

Two whole *Kochers* (clamps to place on the umbilical cord).

Two scissors (a bent one for cutting the umbilical cord, and another type to use if an episiotomy has to be performed).

Box or tin with suturing equipment (various types of thread: self-absorbing for internal use and nylon for external use), two pincettes, needles, scissors, and needleholder.

Mucus extractor for the baby.

Sterile gloves to perform an internal examination.

Sterile gloves to use when the baby is being born.

Resuscitation and oxygen for the baby.

Baby scale.

Medicine:

Oxytoxin ampules for the mother in case of profuse bleeding after the birth.

Methergin ampules (to stop the bleeding after the placenta is shed).

Needles and syringes to inject the above medication.

Vitamin K for the baby (prophylactic, only used for infants that are breastfed).

49. List of articles the mother must have for the birth (the list is put out by midwives):

A thermometer

A small bottle of alcohol (70%)

Two boxes of sterile gauze (16s)

Umbilical bandages or an umbilical clip

Sanitary towels

Zigzag cottonwool

Six absorbent mats

Tape

Some large underpants

A pack of trash bags

A rubber hot water bottle

A large metal hot water bottle

50. In 1991, ultrasound equipment was available in 10 percent of all Dutch midwives' practices (information given by *Nederlandse Organisatie van Verloskundigen*).

51. *See* the review article by Virginie Ringa, Beatrice Blondel, and Gerard Breart, "Ultrasound in obstetrics: do the published evaluative studies justify its routine use?" *International Journal of Epidemiology* 18, 3 (1989): 489–497.

52. de Reu, P.A.O.M., "Routinematige toepassing van de echoscopie in de fysiologische zwangerschap," *Tijdschrift voor Verloskundigen* 12 (1987): 11–15.

53. This is the thesis of Katz Rothman's book *The Tentative Pregnancy, Prenatal Diagnosis and the Future of Motherhood* (New York: Penguin Books, 1987).

54. Meijer, W. J., "Hoe veilig is veilig en hoe zeker is zeker," *Tijdschrift voor Verloskundigen* 12 (1987): 25–28.

55. Cuppen, A., "Goede verloskunde zonder routine echoscopie," *Tijdschrift voor Verloskundigen* 12 (1987): 19–24.

56. Meijer, p. 28.

57. Van der Hulst.

58. Jordan explains that the early "forceps" consisted of only one blade and must have been totally ineffectual. Jordan, Brigitte, "Technology and the social distribution of knowledge: issues for primary health care in developing countries," in *Anthropology and Primary Health Care*, Jeannine Coreil and J. D. Mull (eds.), (Boulder: Westview Press, 1990): 98–120, note 14: 116–117.

59. Katz Rothman, Barbara, *In Labor, Women and Power in the Birthplace* (New York: W. W. Norton & Company, 1982).

60. Katz Rothman, *Recreating Motherhood, Ideology and Technology in a Patriarchal Society* (New York: W. W. Norton & Company, 1989).

61. World Health Organization, *Having a Baby in Europe* (Copenhagen: World Health Organization, 1985).

62. Klinkert.

9

Maternity Home-Care Assistant: A Unique Occupation

Edwin R. van Teijlingen

Pregnancy, labor, and the postnatal period are in principle physiological events, and it is safe to have a delivery that is expected to proceed normally at home.[1]

INTRODUCTION

The Dutch obstetric system is often held up as an example of how the maternity services in other industrialized countries could be improved. Campaigners for maternity services that put women center-stage all cite the Dutch model of maternity care as the ideal for normal pregnancies. Among such proponents are obstetricians[2] and midwives,[3] as well as childbirth activists,[4] researchers,[5] and consumer groups.[6]

The general idea behind this model is that a healthy woman does not need a hospital delivery or a number of days of nursing in a hospital after the birth of her child. It is considered important that a woman has help at home through the early days of the baby's life, as well as information and advice about infant care. Thus, attention is given to the practical needs of all pregnant women, as well as to the medical needs of special cases, such as difficult deliveries and emergencies.

MATERNITY HOME-CARE ASSISTANTS

A key person in this system is the maternity home-care assistant,[7] or *kraamverzorgende*. She assists the midwife or family doctor during deliveries,

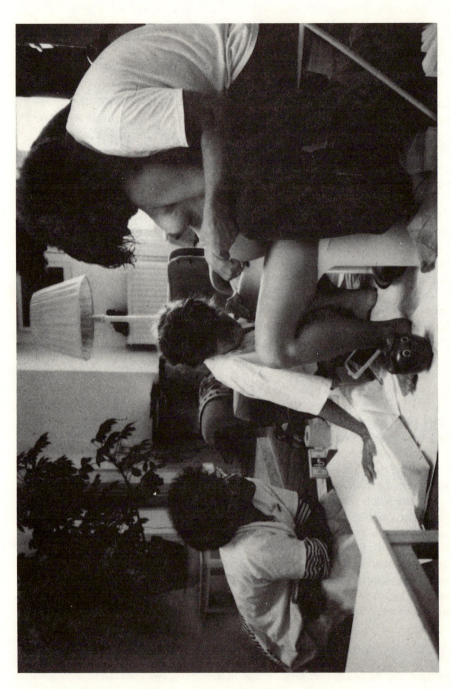

Woman in labor on birthing stool, supported by husband, midwife, and maternity home care assistant. Photo by Astrid Limburg. Used by permission of Astrid Limburg.

and looks after the mother and baby for eight days following the birth if the lying-in period is spent at home. Apart from taking care of the mother and baby, she provides health education, contacts the midwife or family doctor if necessary, looks after other children in the family, does the housework, and may even walk the family dog.

Sheila Kitzinger[8] has written that this unusual occupation does not exist anywhere else in the world. She adds: "It is an important part of the home-birth system in the Netherlands and one without which the midwife would be occupied with simple nursing tasks instead of concentrating on midwifery."[9]

However, Kitzinger's remark needs further substantiation. Some Western countries do provide a similar form of postpartum care, although this is not as comprehensive as in the Netherlands. It does not cater to the majority of healthy new mothers, according to Jo Garcia, Beátrice Blondel, and Marie J. Saurel-Cubizolles (1989): "British women do receive 'home helps' in exceptional circumstances, such as multiple births."[10] Frances V. Price [1990: 139] found in a study of triplets and higher order births in England and Wales in the early 1980s that "all but one household with quadruplets and 61 percent of the households with triplets were provided with at least some support from a local authority home help. In the majority of cases the time allocated to these households was spent doing cleaning, hoovering and ironing."[11] Thus, help that is available only in exceptional cases in Britain is widely available in the Netherlands for normal healthy mothers and their babies, and extends beyond mere house cleaning.

The idea of trained care for the new mother and baby in their own home is not a recent one: maternity home-care assistance courses were initiated around the turn of the century. The first course was established in 1899 in Langedijk, a small town near Amsterdam, and others followed soon after, for example, in Amsterdam (1907) and The Hague (1916).[12] The training of professional assistants for the lying-in period was organized in an attempt to reduce the high infant mortality rates through the instruction of new mothers in the field of health education, hygiene, and baby care.

Relatively late industrialization towards the end of the nineteenth century led to a rapidly expanding population in the urban centers. Because of urbanization, some families lost their traditional kinship networks that provided help during the lying-in period. Moreover, at the end of the century, many midwives wanted to concentrate on their medical tasks and leave the care of mother and infant to others, such as nurses or maternity home-care assistants. These maternity home-care assistants were especially trained to assist midwives attending women of the lower classes and to provide help after the delivery.[13]

The Netherlands was not alone in its attempts to make postnatal care available to new mothers in the first half of the twentieth century. Margaret Dexter and Wally Harbert emphasized that "there have been remarkable parallels in the ways in which home help services have emerged and developed" in different European countries.[14] The first paid home help service started in Germany in 1893 and in England one year later. In 1894, the Sick Room Help Society was established in East London to undertake "household duties where the mother was confined or sick. During pregnancy mothers contributed a small weekly sum for the provision of service for two weeks during confinement."[15]

In Britain, further demands for the provision of help similar to that of maternity home-care assistants, especially for working-class women, followed. "The need for home helps was recognized in all quarters, but wages were poor and suitable workers hard to find," according to Jenny Carter and Thérèse Duriez.[16] Jane Lewis points out that "even with the low wages the helps received, the mothers could not easily afford them."[17]

"Many working-class women preferred to be at home for births after the first because of the difficulty in caring for other children. Women's groups realized this and pointed out the need to include provision for home-helps in any maternity scheme."[18] Jane Lewis also quotes a women's organization, which stated in 1917, that "in the opinion of working women themselves one of their most pressing wants is for reliable help in the home . . . during confinements."[19] However, the organization of such a service was left to local authorities, "who allocated the service very little money in their budgets."[20] The result in Britain was a poor service that varied a great deal from one area to another.

In 1926, the Dutch Ministry of Health laid the foundations of the present maternity home-care organization by establishing training, introducing legislation to protect the occupation, and making it compulsory for maternity home-care assistants to join the local maternity center.[21] The government not only played a major role in establishing the present structure of the organization in the 1940s, but also provided subsidies from 1946 to 1966, when maternity home-care assistance became part of the health insurance system. Legislation and subsidies together played an important role in the rapid expansion of the maternity home-care organization.[22] Currently, the government has an indirect influence through legislation and through its funding of training courses.

Today, the Dutch government promotes home birth attended by midwives or family doctors; its policy is to move care out of the hospital into the home. In a recently published report, the Ministry of Welfare, Health and Culture outlines the policy of "maintaining the quantity and quality of the maternity home-care assistant service, which forms a cornerstone for the whole policy of maintaining or extending the number of home deliveries."[23]

The Parliamentary Committee for Health Care met the secretary of state for Welfare, Health and Culture in December 1989. At this meeting, all the major political parties, from the Left to the Right, agreed that the midwife was the obvious person to provide maternity care, and that deliveries should preferably take place at home.[24] The same secretary of state recognized that home birth depends to a large degree upon the existence of a system of maternity home-care assistance. Moreover, Hans Simons[25] added, the Dutch system is cheaper[26] than that of its neighbors. Fewer obstetricians attending births and more deliveries and postnatal care at home must appeal to governments of industrialized countries trying to cut down their spending on health care.

Work and Training

The duties of maternity home-care assistants are:

1. Assisting a midwife or family doctor during home birth or a short-stay hospital delivery (maximum stay of twenty-four hours)
2. Attending and caring for mother and baby, and looking after any older children in the family
3. Recognizing symptoms in mother and baby that make it necessary to contact the midwife or doctor
4. Providing health education for parents, such as guidance on how to establish breast-feeding or on how to bottle feed the baby, how to change diapers, and information concerning the general health-care of babies
5. Housekeeping and other domestic tasks, such as cooking for the family.

Midwives Beatrijs Smulders and Astrid Limburg state that maternity home-care assistants relieve midwives of the postdelivery nursing activities.[27] For Dutch midwives, postnatal care takes less of their time than it does for British community midwives, because the maternity home-care assistant sees the new mother and baby each day during the lying-in period. The midwife calls in daily after the delivery for four days and then every second day of the lying-in period. If the maternity home-care assistant is not happy about the condition of baby or mother, she contacts the midwife.

In the past two decades the advantages of breast-feeding have been emphasized by researchers, the World Health Organization, Health Ministries, and campaign groups, such as La Leche League International and The National Childbirth Trust (NCT).

The percentage of mothers breast-feeding can be regarded as an indicator of the effectiveness of the health education aspect of the work of maternity home-care assistants. In 1987, 67.4 percent of the mothers who used the service were breast-feeding on the day the maternity home-care assistants left. After an increase in this percentage in the early 1980s, the 1987 figure showed a 1.7 percent decrease compared with the 1986 figure.[28] A Dutch voluntary organization promoting breast-feeding (Borst Voeding Natuurlijk) criticized measuring the breast-feeding rate so soon after delivery. The maternity home-care assistant does a good job stimulating breast-feeding, but what happens when she leaves after eight or ten days? According to a committee member[29] of this organization: "Many women give up after the maternity home care assistant has left. A mother still needs support in her effort to breast-feed her baby after the lying-in period has finished."

In some industrialized countries, this task is performed by breast-feeding counselors, often working for voluntary organizations. La Leche League International, which started in the United States in the mid-1950s and currently has branches all over the world including the Netherlands, provides such information and support. The National Childbirth Trust in Britain has some 500 breast-feeding counselors;[30] these are volunteers who receive an eighteen-month training course in their spare time.[31] By contrast, some hospitals in Britain have gone in the opposite direction by appointing a midwife who is solely employed as breast-feeding counselor. This concern about breast-feeding in itself is praiseworthy. It is, however, questionable whether the person to do this job needs to be a highly trained and relatively expensive midwife.

In general, social and professional distance between mother and maternity home-care assistant will be considerably less than between patients and doctors. Maternity home-care assistants have described the closeness of the relationship between them and the new mothers as follows: "The mothers often ask or tell us things which they do not discuss with their own husband."[32]

Until 1987, maternity home-care assistant training consisted of four months' formal instruction and an apprenticeship of one year under the supervision of an established assistant. Because of cuts in the health services, radical changes have occurred in this training. What had once been a specific course for this work has now been combined with training for a range of community-care work, including general home help, caring for old people, caring for children, and caring for the mentally handicapped.[33]

The employment conditions of maternity home-care assistants are not very generous. Moreover, these women find it hard to combine their irregular working hours with running their own households.[34] They are another example of female providers of health care concentrated in the lower-paid, lower-status jobs.[35]

Dutch maternity centers face problems in recruiting and keeping staff. It is difficult to attract women to take the training course and, more importantly, to take a job as maternity home-care assistant after having taken the course. At the same time, there is a high turnover: 15 percent annually.[36] Most maternity home-care assistants stop working when they have their own children, although some may later return as supply workers.[37]

Since the Netherlands has a rapidly growing immigrant population, maternity home-care assistants have to pay special attention to different cultures. They have to deal with large numbers of women from ethnic minority groups.[38]

ORGANIZATION

Maternity home-care is provided by seventy-six regional and local maternity centers,[39] employing about 3,200 full-time and 1,900 part-time maternity home-care assistants. All but one are women, and about a third of them are employed as "supply" workers, that is, they are called upon to cover for temporary vacancies.[40] The centers are run by the National Cross Organization,[41] which is an autonomous institution for community health care and funded on a fee-for-service basis.

The maternity centers offer three possible arrangements for maternity care: full-time, part-time, and a combination of the two. The favorite service is full-time care; over two-thirds (66.8 percent) of all customers use this type of care. In this arrangement, the maternity home-care assistant stays with the family for eight to ten days.

The second type of care provided by the maternity centers is part-time help, which 14.6 percent of all clients receive.[42] Under this scheme, the maternity home-care assistant visits the mother and child twice a day, usually for an hour and a half in the morning and one hour in the afternoon. Attention is focused on nursing mother and child, and the family is expected to take care of the housework.[43]

Some maternity centers have introduced a combination of the two types of care. This is received by 18.7 percent of all clients.[44] Full-time and part-time care are combined in such a way that they come closer to fulfilling the needs of individual clients. The way in which flexible care is provided varies, since each center operates autonomously.[45]

The percentage of families who make use of maternity home care has increased rapidly over the past ten years, and currently stands at 73 percent of all births, that is to say, about 136,000 births per year.[46] In the larger municipalities (>100,000 inhabitants), maternity home care is provided less frequently than in the smaller towns.[47] This may be explained by a shortage of staff in some larger cities.

A pregnant woman who wants to use the service of a maternity home-care assistant has to apply at the local or regional maternity center. During her first prenatal visit to the midwife (or family doctor), she will be provided with information about this service.[48] Jetske Spanjer et al. (1986) stress that women need to book well in advance.[49] It is virtually impossible to book a maternity home-care assistant after the third month of pregnancy.

The maternity centers try to ensure continuity of care. However, planning is difficult, since it is impossible to predict the number of babies born in a given area on a given day. The expected date of delivery is not a precise indicator, since only 4 percent of all babies are born on this date.

Government cuts in spending on the maternity service mean that maternity centers have to budget for about 15 percent part-time care to reach the average of sixty-four hours of care per family. This implies that many families will be faced with a change of maternity home-care assistant. Maternity home-care assistants also miss out in this situation, being required to work with more families for a shorter period of time.[50] Because of this, they have less opportunity to get to know the parents.[51]

CONCLUDING REMARKS

Maternity home-care assistants play a key role in the low-technology approach of the Dutch maternity services. The very fact that this occupation exists makes it possible for pregnant women in all social classes to opt for a home birth or a short-stay hospital delivery. The assistants provide the new mother with an extra pair of hands and practical knowledge at a special time in her life, as well as helping her in coming to terms with the new baby.

Since the 1980s, the maternity home-care assistant has been the victim of several cuts in government spending. Low wages and social and psychological demands of the job have also led to a shortage of women taking up this occupation, especially in the larger cities. This is an issue that the Dutch have to address now, since the encroachment of the provision of maternity home-care could directly undermine the existing organization of maternity care. To safeguard home delivery, the maternity home-care assistant is indispensable.

NOTES

The author would like to thank Teresa and Peter McCaffery, Graham Barry, Nina Giles, and Annette Ross for all the help and encouragement they have given. This chapter is an edited and modified version of the paper, "The profession of maternity home care assistant and its significance for the Dutch midwifery profession," *International Journal of Nursing Studies*, 27 (1990): 355–66.

1. Ziekenfondsraad, *De Verloskundige Indicatielijst.* (Amstelveen, Ziekenfondsraad, 1987).

2. Rickford, F., "Deliverance," *Marxism Today*, 10 (June 1986): 40.

3. Newson, Katherine, "Direct entry method of training midwives in three countries: 1. The Netherlands," *Midwives Chronicle & Nursing Notes* (Feb. 1981): 39–43.

4. Arms, Suzanne, *Immaculate Deception. A New Look at Women and Childbirth* (3rd ed.) (New York: Bantam Books, 1981).

5. Tew, Marjorie, *Safer Childbirth? A Critical History of Maternity Care* (London: Chapman and Hall, 1990).

6. AIMS (Association for the Improvement of Maternity Services), *Choosing a Home Birth* (leaflet) (London: AIMS, 1986).

7. The fact that there is no equivalent for *kraamverzorgende* in English-speaking countries has led to a confusing variety of English translations: maternity aid nurses, maternal home help, maternity helper, maternity home-care auxiliary nurses, maternity home helps, maternity nurses, and maternity welfare worker. The current translation of maternity home-care assistant, avoiding the confusing usage of the word

nurse, was proposed by Knoop, A., "Letter to editor," *Tijdschrift voor Verloskundigen*, 13 (June 1988): 217–218.

8. Kitzinger, Sheila, *Birth at Home* (Oxford: Oxford University Press, 1980).

9. Ibid., p. 47.

10. Garcia, Jo, Beátrice Blondel, and Marie J. Saurel-Cubizolles, "The needs of childbearing families: social policies and the organization of health care," in *Effective Care in Pregnancy and Childbirth*. Vol. 1, Chalmers, Ian, Murray Enkin, and Marc J. Keirse (eds.) (Oxford: Oxford University Press, 1989).

11. Price, Frances V., "Who helps?" in *Three, Four and More: A Study of Triplet and Higher Order Births*, Botting, Beverley J., Alison J. Macfarlane, and Frances V. Price (eds.) (London: HMSO, 1990): 139.

12. Verbrugge, Hans P., *Kraamzorg bij Huisbevallingen. Evaluatie van Resultaten* (Groningen, Wolters-Noordhoff, 1968): 7.

13. Goote, Helen, *Van Bakerhulp naar Verzorgende: Een Beeld van de Kraamverzorgstersopleiding* (Bunnik: Nationale Kruisvereninging, 1988): 10.

14. Dexter, Margaret, and Wally Harbert, *The Home Help Service* (London and New York: Tavistock Publications, 1983): 1.

15. Ibid., pp. 6–7.

16. Carter, Jenny and Thérèse Duriez, *With Child: Birth Through the Ages* (Edinburgh: Mainstream Publishing, 1986): 140.

17. Lewis, Jane, *The Politics of Motherhood: Child and Maternal Welfare in England, 1900–1939* (London: Croom Helm, 1980): 131.

18. Ibid., p. 130.

19. Ibid., p. 131.

20. Carter and Duriez, p. 140.

21. Verbrugge, p. 9.

22. Ibid., chapter 10.

23. Adviescommissie Verloskunde, *Verloskundige Organisatie in Nederland: Uniek, Bewonderd en Verguisd* (Eindrapport). (Rijswijk: Ministry of Welfare, Health and Culture, 1987).

24. Tweede Kamer der Staten Generaal, *Vaststelling van de begroting van de uitgaven en de ontvangsten van hoofdstuk XVI (Ministerie van Welzijn, Volksgezondheid en Cultuur) voor het jaar 1990*. Tweede Kamer 1989–1990, 21 300 XVI, No. 42, (The Hague: SDU Uitgeverij, 1990).

25. Simons, Hans, "De Verloskundige: Spil of Speelbal?" in *De Vroedvrouw, de Spil van de Verloskunde*, van der Hulst, L. A. M. (Bilthoven: Catharina Schrader Stichting, 1991): 20.

26. The organization of maternity home care is now completely self-financing. The state insurance funds' contribution covers 70 percent of the total costs, the private health insurance companies reimburse 20 percent, and the users of the service contribute 10 percent; *see* Daemers, Marie, and Anne van der Wal, "Structuur, Organisatie en Financiering van de Kraamzorg," *Tijdschrift voor Verloskundigen*, 15 (December 1990): 371–374. Parents have to pay a fee, which varies from about $8 per day for part-time help (16.20 Dutch guilders) to about $20 per day for full-time help (40.50 guilders). The state insurance funds or private insurance companies pay the remaining costs, which vary between $50 daily for part-time help (96.20 guilders) and $122 daily for full-time help (240.50 guilders). Most private health in-

surance companies have similar arrangements for their clients. People on state benefits fall under an exemption, which limits payment for all medical costs to a maximum of $86 (171 guilders) per year. Thus, their maximum contribution is $86, depending on the other medical costs they have incurred that year, according to Zaken, Sociale, *Algemene Bijstandswet. Hoofdlijnen en Bedragen* (leaflet Dutch DHSS), Ministry of Social Security and Employment, The Hague (1 July 1987).

27. Smulders, Beatrijs, and Astrid Limburg, "Obstetrics and midwifery in the Netherlands," in *The Midwife Challenge*, Kitzinger, Sheila (ed.) (London: Pandora Press, 1988).

28. Nationale Kruisvereniging, *Jaarreportage Kraamzorg Kruiswerk 1987* (Bunnik: Nationale Kruisvereniging, 1989).

29. Personal communication from committee member of Borst Voeding Natuurlijk (Breast-feeding Naturally).

30. MIDIRS, *What Is the National Childbirth Trust?* MIDIRS Information Pack, No. 12 (Bristol: MIDIRS, 1989).

31. Personal communication from Dr. Maureen Porter, National Childbirth Trust's breast-feeding counselor in Aberdeen and social researcher in the field of maternity care.

32. Scheijmans, Inge, "De Positie van Vrouwelijke Werknemers in de Kraamzorg," in *Kenau of Nachtegaal, Vrouwen in de Verpleging en Verzorgende Beroepen*, Kroef, Marja, Ineke Jansen, and Nel Willekens (eds.), (The Hague, Ministry Social Security and Employment, 1986).

33. Kiers, J. "Nieuwe Opleiding MDGO-VZ Is Even Wennen!" *MGZ*, 14, No. 9 (1986): 18–19.

34. Bureau Obelon, "Naar een klantgerichte kraamzorg," *Tijdschrift voor Verloskundigen*, 11 (May 1986): 141–154.

35. Abbott, Pamela, and Claire Wallace, *An Introduction to Sociology; Feminist Perspectives* (London: Routledge, 1990): 111.

36. Roumen, Madeleine, *Rotterdams Nieuwsblad* (January 17 1987): 3.

37. Seysener, Mariëtte, and Jancees van Westering, "Kraamzorg in Moeilijke Hoek, Maar Situatie is Niet zó Alarmerend!" *MGZ*, 14 (September 1986): 12–14.

38. Smeenk, Irma, "Werken bij 'n Buitenlands Gezin Vereist Nogal wat Aanpassing," *MGZ*, 14 (September 1986): 23–24.

39. CBS, "Data on Staff of Maternity Centers, 1988," *Maandbericht Gezondheidsstatistiek*, 8 (The Hague: Staatsuitgeverij, 1989): 34–36.

40. CBS, "Data on Staff of Maternity Centers, 1989," *Maandbericht Gezondheidsstatistiek*, 10 (The Hague: Staatsuitgeverij, 1991): 5–7.

41. The National Cross Organization provides the following services:

   a. District nursing: nursing and care for sick and infirm people at home
   b. Centers for infants and toddlers
   c. The provision of health information and education
   d. The loan of medical aids
   e. Prenatal and postnatal care carried out by district nurses and prenatal teachers
   f. Maternity home-care assistance.

42. Nationale Kruisvereniging, 1989.

43. Bureau Obelon, 1986.

44. Nationale Kruisvereniging, 1989.

45. Nationale Kruisvereniging, *Evaluatie Voorbereiding en Invoering Flexibele Kraamzorg tot 1987* (Bunnik: Nationale Kruisvereniging, 1987).

46. Nationale Kruisvereniging, 1989.

47. Ridderbeek, R.J.J., "Deliveries and maternity care, GE 1987/1988," in *Maandbericht gezondheidsstatistiek* 12 (The Hague: SDU/Uitgeverij, 1990): 4–13.

48. Bureau Obelon, 1986.

49. Spanjer, Jetske, et al., *Bevallen en Opstaan* (rev. ed.) (Amsterdam, Uitgeverij Contact, 1986).

50. De Leidster-Docenten van Kraamcentra in de Provincie Zuid-Holland, *Een Zwartboek Over de Kraamzorg* (unpublished), 1987.

51. Ropping, Roelof, "Kraamzorg Drenthe op de Drempel van een Nieuwe Tijd," *MGZ*, 17 (May 1989): 28–29.

10

Illness versus Natural Process: Competing Paradigms in Great Britain and the Netherlands

---

L. H. Lumey

INTRODUCTION

The management of pregnancy, part of a more general debate about the medicalization of society (and of childbirth), is a topic currently discussed by physicians, midwives, sociologists, and the public at large (Freidson, 1975; MacIntyre, 1977). In these discussions, two competing paradigms of pregnancy are put forward. In the first, pregnancy and childbirth are regarded as potentially hazardous diseases that need to be dealt with through medical assistance and intervention. Therefore, deliveries should always take place in a hospital setting. In the second, pregnancy and childbirth are regarded as natural processes in healthy women in whom medical assistance is usually not required. Following this paradigm, most women's deliveries can safely be performed at home. Most Western obstetric systems, including those in Great Britain, are based on the first paradigm. By contrast, the Dutch system is largely based on the second (Torres and Reich, 1989).

The reason given under the first paradigm for concentrating all deliveries in institutions is usually the safety of mother and child. It is not possible to predict that a delivery will be spontaneous and uneventful, argue the proponents of this view, not even when no risk seems to be present: "labor is only normal in retrospect," and labor may suddenly become complicated, calling for specialist services and attention only hospitals can provide. From this perspective, it is better to expose all women to a hospital environment, even if ultimately only a few will need it.

In the Netherlands, however, many people still regard childbirth as a phenomenon not generally calling for intervention by obstetricians unless a complicated delivery is anticipated. It is still accepted that given good prenatal selection of the mothers and ready access to hospital facilities for emergencies, most deliveries can safely be performed by a midwife at home.

These two competing paradigms of pregnancy are illustrated by recent developments in the maternity services of two contrasting systems of obstetric care. The first is in Great Britain, where an interventionist attitude prevails, and the second is in the Netherlands, where a system of home births, mostly attended by midwives, is still prevalent.

The rapid growth of institutional births in Great Britain and the Netherlands is a relatively recent phenomenon. The proportion of home deliveries in England and Wales declined from 85 percent of all births in 1927 to 36 percent in 1958 to 1.1 percent in 1982 (see Figure 1). In the Netherlands, one-third of all births are home deliveries. As late as the early 1960s, 70 percent of all births in the Netherlands still took place at home. After a rapid decline in home births from the mid-1960s to the mid-1970s, the proportion has now stabilized at about one-third of all births (see Figure 2). The transition from home- to hospital-based obstetrics in Western societies started after World War II, continued unabated in the 1950s, and was completed in most countries by the late 1960s. In later sections, we will trace the transition in the activities of the consultative committees on obstetric services in Great Britain and the Netherlands.

HISTORICAL BACKGROUND

Management of Pregnancy before 1900

It was not until the mid-eighteenth century that the first lying-in hospitals for hospital deliveries were founded in England (Donnison, 1977, p. 25). Workhouse infirmaries developed from the 1830s onward. By the end of the nineteenth century, more than 25,000 patients were delivered in twenty-seven London medical charities alone (Van Lieburg and Marland, 1989). In those early days, obstetricians were more concerned about saving the lives of mothers than of babies, since the latter could easily be replaced. In spite of this concern, the practice of institutional confinements was associated with excessive maternal mortality rates many times higher than for home deliveries. There was about one maternal death for every thirty deliveries in institutions in England in the period 1855–67 (McKeown, 1976, p. 105). Similar mortality rates were seen in hospitals all over continental Europe. Hospital confinements were so dangerous to the mother because of the high risks of a puerperal infection. Only the poor, the unmarried, and the homeless delivered in institutions. Maternal mortality and mortality care in the nineteenth century is discussed extensively in a recent monograph (Loudon, 1993).

In the Netherlands, only four lying-in clinics existed by the 1880s. These

Figure 1
Home Births as a Percentage of All Births in England and Wales,
1958–1987

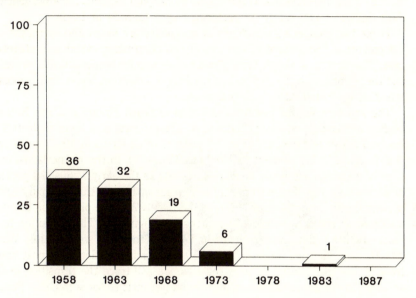

Source: DHSS.

were not an expression of a tendency towards hospital-based childbirth, but were solely a teaching aid for medical students and midwives. The first clinical school for the teaching of medical students was founded in 1828, and the first training school for midwives, a state institution, was begun in 1865. The development of hospital-based obstetrics in the Netherlands was slow, and only a small number of deliveries were handled by obstetricians. By the end of the nineteenth century, the largest clinic in the Netherlands was that of the University of Amsterdam, which saw a maximum of 500 deliveries a year. Nationally, the yearly number of hospital births probably did not exceed 1,000 (Van Lieburg and Marland, 1989). The dangers to the mother of institutional deliveries were well recognized, and it was felt that if at all possible no woman should be subjected to such risks. Births were generally attended by midwives at home.

The Midwives' Role in the Shaping of a Paradigm

As outlined above, the two competing paradigms reflect long-standing differences between the two societies in the management of childbirth. These differences already existed in the last century and have continued ever since. The position of midwives is of particular importance in this context. By the

Figure 2
Home Births as a Percentage of All Births in the Netherlands, 1958–1987

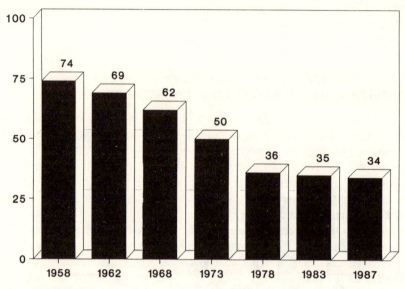

Source: CBS.

turn of this century, the midwives in the Netherlands had established their autonomy in the area of normal childbirth to such an extent that it could not be effectively challenged by the medical profession. The (re)establishment of midwives as "the guardians of normal childbirth" (Marland in this volume) has greatly diminished the medicalization of childbirth in the Netherlands. By the nineteenth century, the division of labor between midwives and doctors ensured that normal deliveries remained within the professional domain of the midwives, while abnormal deliveries were left to physicians. This division of labor would later be supported by midwives, obstetricians, and government alike, and reflects the important position of midwives in the handling of normal deliveries as well as the absence of an expansionist ethos among obstetricians (illustrated by the very low level of institutional deliveries).

These early developments have had a profound effect on the management of childbirth in the twentieth century: The medicalization of childbirth in the Netherlands started much later than in the surrounding countries, and the development towards a general system of hospital deliveries took place at a much slower rate. Normal deliveries in the Netherlands are still mostly handled by midwives, who are independent medical practitioners in the area of obstetrics. It is their responsibility to refer complicated cases to obstetricians for further advice and timely care. Midwives deliver about 45 percent of all infants currently born in the Netherlands (Hessing-Wagner, 1991). Home births assisted by midwives are the continuation of an unbroken tradition in the Netherlands, not a new development as elsewhere. The Dutch paradigm depends on a culture that places a high value on the home, motherhood, and the family, and its consequences on the management of childbirth are felt to the present day.

STATE COMMITTEES ON MATERNITY SERVICES: AN ILLUSTRATION OF COMPETING PARADIGMS

The two paradigms should be seen as outcomes of professional rivalries and state interventions. The State can provide additional support for the prevailing paradigm. Reports of various government committees set up in Great Britain and the Netherlands since the 1950s to evaluate the maternity services and provide guidelines for obstetric practice reflect the developments. In both countries, there was a strong tendency towards maternity services with home and hospital deliveries under unified control, but the contrasting outcomes in the two countries resulted from differences in professional power among the midwives. By 1970 the case load of an average domiciliary midwife in England and Wales had declined to about twenty-five deliveries per year (DHSS, 1970), whereas her Dutch colleague still attended well over 100 (NRV, 1972). In the 1960s and 1970s, a strong hospital service dominated by obstetricians was created in Great Britain. It employed many midwives and left increasingly less space for home deliveries. The independent midwives and active government support in the Netherlands maintained a balance between home and hospital deliveries.

What caused the two vastly different paradigms of childbirth to develop in countries that are geographically so close together and at first sight seem culturally so similar? What caused the management of pregnancy and childbirth to develop so differently in the two highly industrialized societies in which there are so many other areas of broad agreement on medical matters? Cannot scientific medicine give us clear guidelines for managing pregnancy and childbirth, and should not these guidelines be valid for all times and places and be universally implemented? We will draw on the English and Dutch experiences to examine these issues. The discussions within the government committees set up in the two countries to evaluate the obstetric services illustrate that the competing paradigms of pregnancy are an example of the interplay between science and culture and the fact that culture in this confrontation may well be the dominating influence.

On the whole, the various committees in Great Britain and the Netherlands seem to have been selected to support the national paradigm. The committees used the available medical evidence selectively, that is, to support their own beliefs. This was possible because existing national data on perinatal mortality and other outcomes by place of birth are derived from highly selected patient groups and are difficult to interpret: the selection criteria are not adequately documented at the individual level. This leaves much room for speculation. In general, the discussions extolled the virtues of the prevailing national system without critically examining alternative systems, illustrating the extent to which the practice of medicine must be understood in interaction with more general belief systems prevailing in a particular culture.

THE DEVELOPMENT TOWARDS UNIVERSAL HOSPITAL CARE IN GREAT BRITAIN

The Guillebaud Committee

The Beveridge Report of 1942 estimated that a national health service for Great Britain might cost about £170 million a year; other government estimates before 1948 were around the same mark. In fact, in its first full year, the National Health Service (NHS) cost £402 million, more than twice what had been expected (Watkin, 1975).

The extent of the miscalculation shocked the Labour government, which had started the National Health Service, and the error was immediately seized upon by the Conservative opposition. In 1951, the Conservatives won the general election, but they, too, were unable to control the rising costs of the service. Consequently, in 1953, a committee was appointed to look into the costs of the National Health Service. The committee, chaired by C. W. Guillebaud, reported in 1956.

It found that the cost of the NHS, adjusted for population increases, did not actually rise between 1949–50 and 1953–54. No major change was recommended in the general administrative structure of the NHS, but it was noted that the division of the health services into separate branches (i.e., hospital authorities, local executive councils, and local health authorities) had particularly affected the maternity and child welfare services, and that there were wide variations in the provision of these services among local areas (Min. of Health, 1956, paras. 631–632). The Royal College of Obstetricians and Gynaecologists, in particular, felt that the division "tends to produce an atmosphere of competition not cooperation between the various components of the service." Not only the division of services, but also the relation between midwives and doctors had changed with the advent of the National Health Service. The position of the midwife had been seriously weakened, since a midwife attending a delivery in which a doctor was also present was no longer in charge. Further, patients gained direct access to doctors for pregnancy care "not only when the midwife arranged it." These arrangements seriously affected the midwives' control over pregnancy care (Oakley, 1984).

It is clear that the obstetricians wanted unified control of the obstetric services on a regional level, presumably with themselves in command. This could also bring maternity services under control of a single authority to secure a proper balance between the institutional and domiciliary confinements. Just what this proper balance was would be difficult to determine, since the proportion of hospital deliveries varied between 45 and 80 percent by region. According to the committee, 50 percent would represent an adequate provision for hospital confinements in most areas. (This was close to the national average at the time.) As could have been anticipated, the Royal College of Obstetricians and Gynaecologists insisted that "institutional confinement provides the maximum safety for mother and child, and therefore the ultimate aim should be to provide obstetric beds for all women who need or will accept institutional confinement" (Min. of Health, 1956, paras. 633–635).

The Guillebaud Committee suggested that an inquiry into the maternity services be held to suggest more efficient forms of provision (Min. of Health, 1956, para. 693). Because of this recommendation, the Committee on Maternity Services (the Cranbrook Committee) was appointed in April 1956 "to review the present situation of the maternity services in England and Wales, to consider what should be their content and to make recommendations."

The Cranbrook Committee

The committee reported in 1959, and outlined the views of proponents and opponents of home and hospital confinements (Min. of Health, 1959, 17–29). It was clear that the trend towards hospital deliveries had been very pronounced over the preceding twenty-five years, and that, for instance, the United States, Sweden, Australia, and New Zealand were now heading for a universal hospital delivery system. England and Wales were still lagging behind in this respect.

The Royal College of Obstetricians and Gynaecologists reiterated that in their opinion only a hospital confinement could offer maximum safety for the mother and the baby, since even after careful selection, some emergencies do occur in the home. The regional hospital boards and independent women's organizations also noted that there was an unsatisfied demand for hospital confinements in most areas and that beds should be provided for all women who wished to deliver in a hospital. It was argued that women might prefer to have their babies in the hospital, because they thought it was safer, they believed that they could get more complete rest in a hospital, and hospital confinements would be cheaper for the mother.

On the other hand, the Royal College of Midwives and the British Medical Association emphasized some important advantages of home confinements: the fear of labor was diminished in familiar surroundings, and the presence of relatives could be of great help to the mother. Nearly all witnesses recognized that between 10 and 20 percent of the women preferred to have their babies at home, and the College of General Practitioners said that many mothers would prefer home confinement, if assured of its safety.

Several witnesses, including representatives of women's organizations, were of the opinion that the increased demand for hospital confinement was largely due to the interwar propaganda on maternal mortality, and suggested that the death rate now was so low and the advantages of domiciliary confinement so great that active propaganda should be organized to encourage women to have their babies at home if medical and social conditions permitted. This was never adopted as the national policy.

Members of the committee traveled abroad to describe the organization of the maternity services in other countries. One member visiting the Netherlands was surprised to find that in the late 1950s, nearly 80 percent of the confinements in the Netherlands took place at home, that the incidence of breast-feeding there was high (95 percent of babies being breast-fed up to the third month), and that the results obtained within the Dutch system were outstandingly good, with low maternal and perinatal death rates. These results were attributed to the special health and physique of Dutch women and the system of maternity home-care assistants: "In evaluating the success of the Dutch system, the specific cultural and social circumstances of the Netherlands, its semi-rural development and the sense of vocation of Maternity Aids [maternity home-care assistants provided by the state and paid by the patient according to her means] must be taken into account" (Min. of Health, 1959, p. 14). No further elaboration of this issue was given, which suggests that the committee had already made up its mind and wished neither to explore the Dutch situation in more detail nor to assess its relevance for Great Britain.

The committee recommended that facilities should be provided to allow an average of 70 percent institutional confinements in Great Britain, also allowing for most women to stay in the hospital for ten days after delivery. This proportion should cover institutional confinements when an abnormality was present or might be anticipated. It also happened to be close to the proportion of women actually giving birth in hospitals, thus confirming the existing trend.

The committee decided not to urge provision of maternity beds for all confinements, because there would not be enough midwives to staff them; the shortage of practicing midwives was even more acute in the hospitals than in the domiciliary service. There was also a reluctance to use considerably more beds for confinements when other patients might be in more urgent need of hospital facilities.

Between Cranbrook and Peel

The Perinatal Mortality Survey of 1958 that analyzed all births during one week in Great Britain ($n = 17,000$) confirmed that home deliveries were safe for mothers in low-risk categories: infants of mothers booked and delivered at home had a 50 percent lower mortality than the national average. Hospital-booked and delivered births (these include many patients in high-risk categories) had an average mortality figure. Mortality among infants of mothers who had been booked at home but had delivered their babies in a hospital was over three times the national average, however (Butler and Bonham, 1963, pp. 40–42, 52). The particularly high-risk group includes patients originally (i.e., at the beginning of pregnancy) classified as low risk who were later transferred to a hospital because of problems during pregnancy and/or delivery. Some of these patients should have been classified as high risk at the beginning of pregnancy. The survey also suggested that some of the patients had not been booked for a hospital confinement in a timely way. The finding of adverse outcomes in transferred women was used against home deliveries, without further analysis as to whether these women would have fared better had they been booked for a hospital delivery. The fact that many more patients in low-risk categories had not been booked for home confinements and that outcomes in this group could be expected to be very good was never mentioned.

The trend towards hospital confinements was continuing: 65 percent in 1959, the Cranbrook target of 70 percent was reached in 1964, and the national figure in 1969 was over 83 percent (DHSS, 1972, p. 98: Table 15.2) (*see* Figure 1). Under these conditions, it was becoming increasingly difficult to maintain a satisfactory domiciliary midwifery service. The number of home deliveries in England and Wales fell from over 280,000 in 1962 to less than 130,000 in 1969. The only way to prevent unemployment of domiciliary midwives was to assign to them the care of mothers and babies discharged shortly after delivery: the domiciliary midwife was increasingly becoming a maternity nurse for early discharged patients.

Early discharges were mostly a result of the shortage of maternity beds: the number of hospital confinements was growing steadily, while the number of available beds increased much more slowly (DHSS, 1970, p. 67: Tables 1–3). A review of the maternity services to consider the future of domiciliary midwifery and bed needs for maternity patients was urgently required.

The Peel Committee

In the Peel Report of 1970, full institutionalization of childbirth was recommended. This was not surprising, since both the incoming and the outgoing presidents of the Royal College of Obstetricians and Gynaecologists were members of the committee. The Central Midwives Board was represented by its chairman, who happened to be a male physician. The sole female representatives were the president of the Royal College of Midwives and one of her colleagues—clearly not enough to affect the outcome. The government had no intention of deviating from its policy of universal institutional deliveries in setting up this new advisory committee, but it could not ignore the midwives altogether. The obstetricians' argument for institutional confinements was the same as before: "the greater safety for hospital confinements for mother and child justifies the objective of providing sufficient hospital facilities for every woman who desires or needs to have a hospital confinement" (DHSS, 1970, p. 60).

Support for hospital deliveries is provided by a table showing that between 1955 and 1968 maternal mortality rates fell from .59 to .24 per 1,000 births, and perinatal mortality rates fell from 37 to 25 per 1,000 live births, whereas in the same period, the percentage of confinements in institutions increased from 64 to 81 percent of all deliveries (DHSS, 1970, Table 5). One observer remarked that every public health student knows that this sort of correlation is not evidence (Cochrane, 1971, p. 63), because correlation does not imply causation. A similar correlation might have been observed between the increasing number of automobiles and the decreasing perinatal mortality over that period.

The Central Midwives Board did not think that a 100 percent hospital delivery over the country would ever be achieved and "were satisfied that in all areas there will be a continuing need for midwives to be available for domiciliary deliveries" (DHSS, 1970, p. 121). One feels that the majority of the Peel Committee would have preferred to ban domiciliary confinements altogether and that only the fear of a violent reaction from midwives prevented this: "Only a minority of women choose home confinement but we accept the view of the Royal College of Midwives and Chairmen of local Medical Committees that wishes for home confinement should be respected provided, of course, that there are no medical or social contra-indications" (DHSS, 1970, p. 54). Again, home deliveries are defined as the deviation from the norm; contraindications to hospital deliveries are never considered. Since the proportion of women delivering in hospitals had already risen considerably in the absence of specific policy directions and showed no signs of levelling off, the committee recognized "that the discussion of the advantages and disadvantages of home or hospital deliveries is in one sense academic." It was sanctioning developments that had largely taken place already outside its sphere of influence.

The committee also recommended that the maternity services be unified under a single authority. Obstetricians, general practitioners, and midwives should work in teams to provide medical and midwife care, and the local authorities should make arrangements with hospitals to provide a domiciliary maternity service, insofar as such a service was still required. This would enable all midwives to be employed by the hospitals.

The recommendations of the Peel Committee were pre-empted by the 1974 reorganization of the National Health Service, which brought all midwives under the same employers who were health authorities, not hospitals. In most places community midwives maintained a separate identity, although mainly performing postnatal rather than delivery care (Alison Macfarlane, personal communication).

THE DEVELOPMENT TOWARDS INCREASED HOSPITAL CARE IN THE NETHERLANDS: NO LOSS OF THE HOME DELIVERY SYSTEM

The 1972 Report on the Provision of Obstetric Services

In 1966, it had become clear that perinatal mortality rates in the Netherlands were no longer the lowest in the world. This affected national pride, since it had always been taken for granted that the Dutch system of delivering babies at home by midwives was the best. It was not clear, however, if the reason for the Netherlands falling behind was its reluctance to opt for the system of universal hospitalized childbirth. Should the Netherlands retain its system of selection for planned home and hospital deliveries, or had the time come to rethink the organization of obstetric services (Kloosterman, 1966)? In 1963, about two-thirds of all deliveries were still taking place at home, compared to one-third in England and Wales and one in five in Scotland (VOMIL, 1976, p. 10). The high rate of home confinements in the Netherlands had started to drop, however, much as it had previously done in England and Wales. In 1972, only one-half of all deliveries took place at home. Fifteen years earlier, it had been three out of four deliveries (*see* Figure 2). Many reasons for an increase in hospital deliveries can be given: new medical technologies emerged, the number of midwives and physicians (including obstetricians) grew rapidly, and the annual number of births in the Netherlands declined year after year. Competition among health-care providers over fewer births resulted. In addition, hospital births seemed to be the ideal option for those mothers who wanted to avoid all possible risks.

The developments increasingly challenged the prevailing Dutch "home birth" paradigm of pregnancy that for so long had been supported by government, midwives, medical profession, and the lay public alike. These new developments were also proving to be more costly than the traditional arrangements. It is not surprising that the health insurance funds, covering medical expenses for 70 percent of the population in the Netherlands, wanted to know more about the various factors contributing to this trend. Therefore the Central Public Health Council (*Nationale Raad voor de Volksgezondheid NRV*), which includes representatives from the government, the (private) health insurance funds, and the hospitals, appointed a committee that reported its findings in 1972. Although the various British committees were selected to support the prevailing interventionist paradigm, the Dutch committees supported the paradigm of physiological childbirth. This illustrates the preference for home births on the part of government officials and other policy makers in the Netherlands. Within the medical profession itself, many different opinions existed side by side. This is illustrated by the fact that the obstetricians' seat on the committee was taken by Gerrit-Jan Kloosterman, professor of obstetrics at the University of Amsterdam, an esteemed member of the medical establishment, but also late medical director of the state midwife training school in Amsterdam and an eloquent supporter of the midwives' primacy in the area of low-risk deliveries. He had received his professional training at de Snoo's clinic at the University of Utrecht. De Snoo had been in charge of the other midwife training school (in Rotterdam, 1912–26) before he was appointed in Utrecht. Kloosterman has always acknowledged how much he valued de Snoo's noninterventionist approach in the management of childbirth.

The committee estimated that because of the good obstetric outcomes attained under the prevailing system, between 60 and 70 percent of all confinements could safely take place at home (the national figure at the time), provided that adequate prenatal care and selection of patients at risk were guaranteed, and that patients could reach a well-equipped hospital within an hour in case of an emergency. One member of the committee formally objected to the conclusions outlined above and wrote a minority statement advocating universal hospital deliveries. His statement was included in the report but had no response.

Expressing the view that "normal confinements" do not require hospital treatment, the committee also suggested that obstetric centers (verloskundige centra) be started: these would be maternity units staffed by midwives similar to the Zeeburg unit in Amsterdam, which had produced good results between 1948 and 1970 (NRV, 1972). This unit was founded by the city council of Amsterdam to provide facilities for confinements of women with low-risk pregnancies who could not have their babies at home because of poor housing facilities or some other reason. Most patients came from working-class backgrounds. Midwives had overall responsibility for the prenatal, natal, and postnatal care of the women admitted. An obstetrician (a resident from the University of Amsterdam teaching hospital) was required to examine all women at least once during pregnancy, give medical advice at the request of the midwives, and establish criteria for the selection of women at risk. In case of emergency, the midwife in charge could have her patient transferred to the obstetric service of the University of Amsterdam hospital or send for obstetric assistance. If needed, residents would occasionally perform forceps deliveries in the unit. Perinatal mortality in the unit (1948–70) was 7/1,000 in 18,421 births, about three times lower than the national average of 19/1,000 births in the Netherlands in 1970. The reports do not explicitly state whether these statistics excluded women who ended up giving birth in the university hospital because of complications during delivery. These should of course be included for appropriate comparisons.

The Sikkel Committee

In the late 1970s, the increase in hospital deliveries continued. Because many health insurance companies refused to reimburse institutional deliveries (unless a formal medical diagnosis of high-risk pregnancy was made), the rise in institutional deliveries can only be explained by a shift in the application, by obstetricians, of the risk selection procedures: more women than in the past were diagnosed to be at high risk. The shift served both the financial and scientific interests of obstetricians and the interests of those women who wanted a hospital delivery, even if there was no medical need for it. The health insurance funds tried to stem the tide of institutionalized childbirth by threatening to withhold reimbursement of hospital costs in cases where the high-risk criteria had been applied too readily. Short-term hospital deliveries were introduced in 1965. These are hospital deliveries sometimes supervised by midwives or family doctors, with a speedy discharge (less than twenty-four hours) and traditional maternity home-care assistance at home. This intermediary pattern of care combined some advantages of the low- and high-technology obstetric systems. Home-based normal deliveries were still the main characteristic of the Dutch system, but the underlying paradigm was now increasingly being challenged by family doctors and obstetricians. Many of the latter continued to support the old paradigm.

Faced with the new developments and a shift in women's preferences, the Sikkel Committee (1979), chaired by a former Obstetrics Professor of Leiden University, stated its support for home deliveries, and also speculated on the scientific pros and cons of short-term hospital deliveries under the supervision of midwives and family doctors. Because there were no concrete data to evaluate the quality of obstetric care in the Netherlands, speculation was the only possibility. The committee members felt that the new forms of outpatient obstetrics could potentially lead to better collaboration between midwives, family doctors, obstetricians, and pediatricians, and on a much larger scale than was already the case. They also felt that the quality of obstetric care could be improved if competition (for patients and fees) among midwives, family doctors, and obstetricians could be avoided. Therefore, they suggested that any financial arrangements that might favor hospital deliveries be removed.

The committee was also aware of some important administrative and organizational problems that needed to be resolved. For instance, nationally agreed upon rules were needed to ensure access of midwives and family doctors to all obstetric facilities, to ensure uniform procedures for collecting data on pregnancy and delivery, and to define the concepts of low- and high-risk pregnancies. Various agreements relating to these issues needed to be negotiated on a national level among representatives of professional organizations of midwives, family doctors and obstetricians, and hospital boards and the Ministry of Health. A nationwide contract for admission of midwives to all hospitals to perform outpatient obstetrics was agreed upon in 1981. A draft agreement for obstetric centers governing the various professional responsibilities within the hospital setting was agreed upon in 1987. Large sections of this agreement outline arbitration procedures to be invoked in case of professional disagreements and rivalries. In the proposed agreement, family doctors and midwives explicitly retained ultimate responsibility for patients they delivered in a hospital, unless obstetric assistance by hospital staff was explicitly sought. A standard case record form for pregnancy and delivery was agreed upon, and subcommittees were established to revise the definitions of low- and high-risk pregnancies.

A fundamental difference of opinion emerged between the various professional organizations and the Ministry of Health on the one side and the National College of Obstetricians on the other over a revision of the list of indications for institutional deliveries. The settlement of this matter illustrates how much support still existed in the late 1980s for the Dutch paradigm of physiological childbirth.

In an attempt to refine the selection of patients at risk, a new category between the existing low-risk and high-risk categories was introduced. For a patient in this borderline category, the midwife now had to consult with the obstetrician if her patient should be considered at low or high risk during the remainder of the pregnancy. After this consultation, it was up to the midwife to decide if the patient should be referred to an obstetrician for further care. The obstetricians challenged this procedure, and claimed that once a midwife had requested advice, the decision to refer was not hers anymore but theirs. The issue at stake was really the following: should midwives or obstetricians be in charge of patients with borderline risk? In part, this controversy was a fight over patients' fees and dominance in the marketplace, albeit couched in appropriate medical terms referring to the safety of mother and child. It was very clear that the obstetricians received no support from the state or from other parties and would have to give in over time. From within the obstetrical profession, the midwives' position was consistently supported by Kloosterman and fellow obstetricians of the University of Amsterdam medical school. His successor, P. E. Treffers, has continued the department's tradition of support for the midwife as the central provider of prenatal and obstetric care in low-risk pregnancies. Many other academic obstetric departments are more inclined to support interventionist obstetrics.

Ultimately (in 1987), the obstetricians were outvoted by the national providers of health-care insurance, putting the midwife in charge of patients with low and borderline risk. She must refer high-risk cases to the obstetrician in a timely way.

The Kloosterman Committee

The continued decline in home deliveries and the concomitant shift towards high-technology obstetric care provided by obstetricians caused the secretary of health to appoint an expert committee in 1984 to advise him on the organization of obstetric services in the Netherlands. In the best of national traditions, most of the committee members were supportive of the national paradigm of home deliveries for low-risk patients. The committee was chaired by Kloosterman (known from his work on the earlier 1972 committee and among gynecologists as the most outspoken protagonist of "nonmeddlesome midwifery"). It also included three midwives, two general practitioners, and two other gynecologists supportive of the midwives' role. Among the latter was D. van Alten, who had been responsible for setting up a large follow-up study of a cohort of infants mostly delivered by midwives at home. This came to be known as the Wormerveer study, after a small town just north of Amsterdam. Kloosterman had formulated guidelines for hospital referral that had come to be generally accepted for obstetric policy in the Netherlands. His summary of these guidelines runs as follows:

> As a precondition for home confinement now, we ask for the absence of all indications of abnormality. A woman is allowed to stay at home (and is entitled to engage a maternity [home-care assistant] nurse) if she is in good health; if there are no features of toxemia, providing there is no hypertension, if the head of the baby is well engaged, and if there are no symptoms of disproportion. There must not be a multiple pregnancy, nor abnormalities in the medical and obstetrical history. If nulliparous, the woman must be under 35 years of age or if multiparous, under 45 years. Labor must start spontaneously after 38 weeks and before the end of the forty-second week (before 295th day after last menstruation). The social circumstances of the expectant mother must be: a bedroom with heating equipment at her disposal and toilet facilities on the same floor. In case of emergency, there must be the means to transfer her to the nearest hospital within 60 minutes. (Kloosterman, 1978)

The committee members were in basic agreement with the recommendations of the earlier Sikkel Report. They blamed the government for implementing only the Sikkel Committee recommendations that seemed to provide immediate cost savings. Specifically, the government had decided not to reimburse the costs of short-stay hospital deliveries. Members of the Kloosterman Committee feared that by refusing this reimbursement an important opportunity had been lost to stimulate the much-needed improvement in the collaboration among midwives, family doctors, and obstetricians. Since professional rivalries between midwives and obstetricians were still very much in existence, the committee felt that the policy was shortsighted and possibly counterproductive. These professional rivalries must be seen within the context of a very different balance of power in the Netherlands compared to the situation in other countries, since midwives are much more autonomous and powerful in the Netherlands. Money was needed to lower the work load of domiciliary midwives, whose income was based on an estimated number of over 165 deliveries a year.

The Kloosterman Committee recommended that the government provide financial support to midwives, family doctors, and obstetricians to set up integrated services at the local level. Experience with such groups showed that obstetric outcomes in patients were better than average and that a higher proportion of home deliveries supervised by midwives was obtained. It was also felt that priority should be given to systematic documentation of the results obtained by such collaborative efforts, since this would be the only way to show skeptical observers, both inside and outside the country, that the Dutch system of obstetric care could combine high professional standards among those providing the care with a minimum of medical interventions in normal pregnancies. Second, the committee recommended vigorous support of the prevailing system of maternity home-care assistants. Finally, the lack of a comprehensive national data base to document outcomes of pregnancy in home and hospital deliveries was deplored. Without such data, a genuine evaluation of the Dutch system would never be possible.

CONCLUSIONS

The debate about how best to manage pregnancy and delivery, as illustrated by the reports of various advisory committees in Great Britain and the Netherlands, was prompted by contrasting developments in these countries. By comparing maternity services from different regions in Great Britain in the 1950s, wide variations were observed. Since some regions still had relatively high numbers of home deliveries, this was taken by some to indicate that they were lagging behind in quality of care. Especially the Royal College of Obstetricians and Gynaecologists felt that equal quality of care could only be achieved within a system of universal institutional deliveries. In their view, only hospital deliveries could provide optimal safety for mother and child. Such a system was pretty much in place by the early 1980s.

In the Netherlands, by contrast, the state was alarmed when the proportion of home deliveries started to drop rapidly in the 1960s. This decrease was considered undesirable. The fall was in part due to the pregnant women themselves, who increasingly favored short-stay hospital deliveries because these seemed to combine the maximum safety of an institutional delivery with an early discharge home. That home births were also safe was never really challenged, however.

The Dutch paradigm of pregnancy and childbirth and the government response to an increase in hospital deliveries cannot be understood without appreciating the strong position occupied by midwives in the system of maternity care. Midwives have traditionally been responsible for the majority of normal births in the Netherlands because of the relative lack of power of obstetricians. The Dutch paradigm of pregnancy is probably also associated with a national ideology strongly supporting the home, family, and motherhood. To the present day, the Dutch government has supported midwives in their claim that they should have primary responsibility for normal deliveries and that the decision to refer problem cases to obstetricians is theirs alone. In addition, the midwives' position has received considerable support from physicians. Thus, the existence of two vastly different paradigms of childbirth in countries close together geographically and culturally may be explained by the very different position of the midwife in these two countries. In line with the Dutch paradigm of physiologic pregnancy, postpartum care for mothers delivering at home (or discharged early after a short-stay hospital delivery) is given by maternity home-care assistants, a profession not known outside the Netherlands.

The composition of the government committees set up in Great Britain and the Netherlands illustrates that the members were selected to confirm prevailing government policy, without alienating rival professional groups. It is not possible from the published reports to know how this selection was achieved and what compromises, if any, were reached in the selection process. It is obvious, however, that once the members were chosen, the outcome was largely determined. The discussions within the government committees set up to evaluate the obstetric services illustrate that the competing paradigms of pregnancy are an example of the interplay between science and culture and the fact that culture in this confrontation often is the dominant influence.

From an overview of evaluation studies performed in the Netherlands (Treffers et al., 1990), it is becoming increasingly clear that the place of birth is only one of many aspects of Dutch obstetric care that differs from most other Western countries. More comparative studies will need to be done to discover and promote the system of obstetric care that best puts the needs and wishes of pregnant women alongside the advantages provided by medical progress and increasing professional standards. This will be the real challenge for those managing childbirth in the Netherlands now and in the future.

REFERENCES

Butler, N. R., and D. G. Bonham (eds), *Perinatal mortality. The first report of the 1958 perinatal mortality survey.* Edinburgh & London: Livingstone, 1963.

Cochrane, A. L., *Effectiveness and efficiency. Random reflections on health services.* London: The Nuffield Provincial Hospitals Trust, 1971.

Department of Health and Social Security (DHSS), *Domiciliary and maternity bed needs. Report of the Subcommittee of the Standing Maternity and Midwifery Advisory Committee* (Chairman: Sir John Peel). London: DHSS, 1970.

Department of Health and Social Security (DHSS), *Report on Confidential Enquiries into Maternal Deaths in England and Wales 1967–69.* London: DHSS, 1972.

Donnison, Jean, *Midwives and medical men. A history of inter-professional rivalries and women's rights.* London: Heinemann, 1977.

Freidson, Eliot, *Profession on Medicine. A study of the sociology of applied knowledge.* New York: Dodd Mead and Co., 1975.

Hessing-Wagner, J. C., *Geboorte en zorgvernieuwing.* 's-Gravenhage: VUGA, 1991.

Kloosterman, G. J., "De bevalling aan huis en de hedendaagse verloskunde." *Nederlands Tijdschrift voor Geneeskunde* 110 (1966) 1808–1815.

————, "The Dutch system of home births." In Kitzinger, S., and J. A. Davis (eds) *The place of birth*. Oxford: Oxford University Press, 85–92, 1978.

Loudon, I., *Death in childbirth. An international study of maternal care and maternal mortality, 1800–1950*. Oxford: Oxford University Press, 1993.

MacIntyre, S., "The management of childbirth: a review of sociological research issues." *Social Science and Medicine* 11 (1977) 477–84.

McKeown, Th., *The modern rise of population*. London: Edward Arnold, 1976.

Ministry of Health, *Enquiry into the cost of the National Health Service* (Chairman: C. W. Guillebaud). London: HMSO, 1956.

Ministry of Health, *Report of the Committee on Maternity Services* (Chairman: the Earl of Cranbrook). London: HMSO, 1959.

Ministerie van Volksgezondheid en Milieuhygiene (VOMIL), *De verloskundige organisatie in Nederland* (Chairman: A. Sikkel). 's-Gravenhage: VOMIL, 1979.

Ministerie van Volksgezondheid en Milieuhygiene (VOMIL), *Statistische gegevens over de verloskundige organisatie 1960–1974*. Verslagen adviezen en rapporten no. 58, 's-Gravenhage: VOMIL, 1976.

Ministerie van Welzijn, Volksgezondheid en Cultuur (WVC), *Verloskundige organisatie in Nederland: Uniek bewonderd en verguisd*. Eindrapport adviescommissie verloskunde (Chairman: G. J. Kloosterman) VR 87/4. 's-Gravenhage: WVC, 1987.

Nationale Raad voor de Volksgezondheid (NRV), *Advies inzake de verstrekking van verloskundige hulp*. Verslagen en rapporten no. 27. 's-Gravenhage: Ministerie van Volksgezondheid en Milieuhygiëne, 1972.

Oakley, A., *The Captured Womb*. Oxford: Basil Blackwell, 1984.

Torres, A., and Reich, M. R., "The shift from home to institutional childbirth: A comparative study of the United Kingdom and the Netherlands." *International Journal of Health Services*, 19 (1989) 405–14.

Treffers, P. E., Eskes, M., Kleiverda, G., and van Alten, D., "Home births and minimal interventions." *Journal of the American Medical Association*, 264 (1990) 2203–2208.

Van Lieburg, M. J., and Marland, H., "Midwife regulation education and practice in the Netherlands during the nineteenth century." *Medical History* 33 (1989) 296–317.

Watkin, B., *Documents on health and social services, 1834 to the present day*. London: Methuen & Co Ltd., 1975.

11

Interview with Professor Gerrit-Jan Kloosterman

Rineke van Daalen and Reinie van Goor

Gerrit-Jan Kloosterman has an almost legendary reputation, not only in the Netherlands, but also in international circles of obstetricians. He is an obstetrician himself, but he also ardently defends the Dutch obstetric system, with its division between normal deliveries at home attended by midwives and pathological deliveries in hospitals attended by obstetricians. This point of view makes Kloosterman a lonely figure among specialist colleagues abroad and, to a much lesser degree, in the Netherlands, where almost 90 percent of the obstetricians accept his view that healthy women must have a free choice between hospital and home delivery. His advocacy of home birth causes him to be reviled by champions of advanced technology, but makes him a favorite among those who want to improve primary care and preserve home birth and autonomous midwives.

Kloosterman was born in 1915 and completed his medical studies in 1947. In that year, he came to Amsterdam, where he was appointed director of the School for Midwives. Ten years later, he became professor in obstetrics and gynecology at the University of Amsterdam, a position he held until 1983. In the last few years of his professorship, he became increasingly concerned with the Dutch obstetric system, especially in preserving home birth. His concern for good prenatal care to improve ways of screening for low- and high-risk pregnancies is thus quite understandable. His ideas have not only influenced obstetricians and gynecologists in Amsterdam and in the Netherlands in general, but they have also been attended to in other countries. He became Fellow *ad eundem* of the Royal College of Obstetricians and Gynaecologists and Honorary Fellow of the American College of Obstetricians and Gynecologists.

His views are based on trust in nature and respect for the preferences of the woman. The first part, the trust in nature, is allied with great curiosity for the physiology of pregnancy and birth and with a reserved, critical attitude towards new medical inventions and interventions. Respect for the woman's preferences is reflected in Kloosterman's interest in the psycho-social aspects of his profession. This interest manifested itself in attention to the psychosomatic aspects of pain during birth. It has led him to be active in supporting a woman's right to have an abortion since 1967.

BECOMING AN OBSTETRICIAN

I was born in a humanistically oriented family in Arnhem, a town in the eastern part of the Netherlands. I started to study medicine because I was interested in people, the most fascinating and incomprehensible part of Creation. I felt less attracted by studies that dealt only with dead nature. My interest in people had both physical and spiritual aspects. A human being must be perceived as a totality.

Originally I wanted to become a generalist, a general practitioner somewhere in the countryside. That work would give me the opportunity to practice all the different aspects of the study of medicine. Attending at deliveries was at that time an important part of a general practitioner's work. He must be well prepared to give obstetric assistance in rural districts. After completion of my medical study in Utrecht, I decided to spend one year at the university clinic for obstetrics and gynecology (with Professor K. de Snoo). Soon I became so absorbed in that specialty and its scientific aspects that I stayed seven years and became a gynecologist. I wrote my thesis in that field, on the subject of the rhesus factor and polylethality.

IN SUPPORT OF THE MIDWIFE

I came to the School for Midwives not because I loved the midwife, but because I loved the profession. It was my scientific interest that led my teacher to encourage me to apply for the function of Director of the Amsterdam School for Midwives. In those days that position represented a move in the direction of a scientific career. Directors of schools for midwives were "subprofessors," who not only practiced what they had learned at the university, but tried to advance the profession further. I was especially attracted by that combination.

The School for Midwives in Amsterdam was one of the three institutes for the education and training for midwives. These institutes were obstetrical and gynecological hospitals, responsible for more than a thousand deliveries a year and a large number of gynecological operations. Fifty pupil midwives worked for three years as interns in that hospital and attended twenty hours of weekly theoretical and practical instruction in the delivery room, the wards, and the incubator room.

The midwife schools were relatively isolated from obstetric science and had little affiliation with developments in the medical world. I was afraid that this isolation would make them second-rate institutions. In 1956, I suggested to the Amsterdam Municipality that the School for Midwives should be integrated in a well-equipped municipal hospital, but it took twenty years before this integration was finally arranged. Now the schools for midwives in Heerlen and Rotterdam have also been integrated in hospitals. In my opinion, this association with hospitals was their salvation. It is only possible to work at a top level when there are laboratories at your disposal, and when you cooperate with surgeons, specialists for internal diseases, pediatricians, and bacteriologists.

Dutch midwives have kept their relatively strong position because they are legally qualified to practice obstetrics autonomously since the Health Law of 1865. They were never classified as nurses or as paramedical personnel as they are in neighboring countries. At their examination, the Dutch midwives' oath to practice obstetrics to the best of their knowledge and ability is a more restricted version of the one physicians take in medicine, surgery, and obstetrics. The medical world in 1865 was of the opinion that the midwife should not be subordinate to doctors, but should work at their side. She could and can see part of the profession of medicine as her own.

But as prosperity rose and the number of doctors increased, doctors began to take over the work of midwives. They pretended they could do that work better. Some physicians wanted to keep rich patients for themselves and sent the needy ones to the midwife, who became the doctor for the poor. This situation changed in the second half of the twentieth century, at least in the Netherlands. Although it amazed some people, I referred women with a normal pregnancy to a midwife. The wealthy husband of a client whom I referred to a midwife in the 1950s was highly indignant about my advice and cried: "How can I explain to my friends that I send my wife to a midwife? They will think that I try to economize at her expense." Since then I have always stressed the fact that the midwife is not meant as a help to the poor, but as a protector to the healthy.

There have always been people who saw the potential of the midwife, but only in the Netherlands has the potential been realized. We have continually updated the knowledge and experience of the midwife. As far as preventive measures are concerned, we enable midwives to use the most recent advances in obstetric science.

Until the end of the nineteenth century, midwives, like doctors, only attended during the birth. When the importance of prenatal care became clear, midwives also received the right to care for a pregnant woman, first from the twenty-sixth week, later from the start of the pregnancy. Only if there is pathology must a midwife refer clients to an obstetrician.

When I was director of the School for Midwives, I was instrumental in getting the law passed permitting midwives to repair a tear in the perineum. When syphilis tests, blood tests, and rhesus factor tests became part of prenatal care, some people said: "You cannot leave that to midwives." I said: "I do not know any reason why midwives could not perform such tests. Doctors do not test the blood themselves; they, too, send it to a laboratory. It does not make any difference if the sample has been taken by a physician or by a midwife." Actually, there are no scientific or rational arguments for a doctor's monopoly in these respects. In my view, that is only an artificial way of relegating the midwife to a subordinate role. Finally the law was altered in 1955, and some time later, midwives were allowed to give local anesthesia. Whenever advances in knowledge and technology threatened to leave the midwife behind, we adjusted her qualifications so that she had access to all methods of preventive medicine, including ultrasound.

TRUST IN NATURE

Respect for nature, that is characteristic for Dutch obstetrics. The old ideas of Hippocrates about natural healing power are often practiced in the Netherlands, even in obstetrics. "Masterly expectancy" was a typically English catch word, which was very important at a delivery. There were always warnings against impatience. A well-known nineteenth-century German professor, Ahlfelt, recommended to his pupils to leave their forceps at home. If they needed them, they could go home and get them; in the meantime the baby was often born. While this recommendation was given in many nineteenth-century textbooks, in the Netherlands it was really practiced. This trust in nature when dealing with medical issues is an important feature of the Dutch culture.

After World War II this mentality changed, especially under the influence of Western obstetricians who are impressive when handling pathology but sometimes abuse their possibilities. In many highly developed countries, 25 percent of the pregnant women deliver with a Caesarean section, and once a Caesarean section has been done, it often means Caesarean sections for later births. In the Netherlands, this is not necessarily the case. If there is no indication for a Caesarean section in the next pregnancy, the woman will have her baby in the normal way. It can be said that there is a Dutch obstetric tradition in the sense that practicing technology is not that pivotal. An ordinary healthy woman with a normal pregnancy is essentially able to look after herself. We take this as our basic assumption.

In the United States, in Sweden, and in England much effort is devoted to arranging a painless birth. Lately, a group of English members of Parliament visited one of the academic hospitals in Amsterdam. To my great surprise, they suggested that the fact that so many Dutch women had their babies spontaneously, without any anesthesia, was related to our Calvinism. The Calvinist view is to give birth to children in sorrow. The Dutch would keep anesthesia from women in labor because of the Old Testament. That idea never occurred to me before. It is an interesting viewpoint, but it is not mine. It is obvious that we try to make childbirth as pleasant and painless as possible.

I blame many obstetricians who prevent those women willing to accept some hardship to bring forth their children without anesthesia from doing so. When women became aware of the dangers inherent in childbirth as they came to realize that some children were born with a handicap, that stillbirths could happen, and that some women died in childbed, birth became sorrowful, more an emotional than a physical burden. This is also what the Bible says—it does not say that birth became painful: "In sorrow wilt thou bring forth thy children." Other languages use the same word: in German the word is *Beschwer.* I am not a scripturalist, but the image is apt.

Physical pain at childbirth is above all caused by emotions; for that reason a physical approach in fighting pain is not adequate. It is obvious that it is the mission of physicians to lessen pain, but what is the best way to do that during labor? You can make a woman senseless, or you can paralyze her by giving her injections, but these are somatic methods to allay the pain. Once I heard an American midwife say: "Our obstetrics is perineum-centered." That was a good description. Many obstetricians do not look beyond that small part of the body, but many problems in pregnancy, especially during birth, take place in the cerebrum and must be treated there: by helping women in psychic distress, by attending them carefully during pregnancy, and by reassuring them during birth.

THE WOMAN'S WISHES

The wishes of the woman are the only valid argument in obstetrics. Her will must be decisive: if she wants to have birth without any intervention, without anesthesia, without having an episiotomy, if she wants to give birth at home and in the presence of her husband, and if she wants to hold her baby right after birth and to put it to her breast, if there are no medical contraindications, she must be allowed to do so. She also must be free to choose the place of delivery. Financial arguments should not be the main ones in making this choice.

Coercion is wrong under any circumstances. That holds even for abortion. The mother-to-be is the protector of the unborn life, not the physician. If she does not want the baby, it makes no sense to force her. My ideas changed a lot in that respect. I hesitated for a long time, but now I can see abortion as a kind of assistance. At present, I consider my original view, that doctors should protect the unborn life, an overestimation of our own importance, as a masculine attitude that does not do justice to the pregnant woman.

THE NORMAL AND THE PATHOLOGICAL

In our obstetric system, in which patience is so important, midwives are indispensable. Obstetricians who have studied for twelve years at the university are not the right ones to sit next to a woman, hold her hand, and wipe her forehead. A doctor can do that a couple of times, but if that is all he does, he will start to ask himself: "Why did I study?" There is the possibility he will become impatient and irritated, and will think, "The devil, the baby still isn't there. . . . I'll get it." In any case, he uses technology and is admired because of that. "Clever doctor, beautiful forceps, the head of the baby doesn't even show any signs that it was used," or "these Caesarean section babies always have such beautiful round heads. That is nice for these children; they will be clever pupils."

People like to hear what technology can do, and that is the way medicine developed in many countries in the Western world, but medical knowledge has been overrated in the twentieth century. Edward Shorter's *A History of Women's Bodies* demonstrates this overestimation; he sees obstetricians and gynecologists as the liberators of women who were permanently anemic, afflicted with complaints of menstruation, and many dying in childbed. Their feeble constitution made them subordinate to men until gynecologists released them from the vexations of their body. This is such terrible nonsense. At the end of the nineteenth century, during the first wave of feminist emancipation, gynecologists were almost powerless.

After World War II, obstetricians came to have an ever stronger hold on the obstetric system. Up to the 1950s, they were still willing to visit a laboring woman at home, while country doctors were semiobstetricians. The general practitioner dealt with much pathology until the 1960s, but after that time, obstetricians only attended to women in a hospital. During the 1970s, even general practitioners did fewer deliveries. Their experience with home birth was not sufficient anymore because of the declining birth rate. Besides, they did not like to wake up in the middle of the night for a normal birth.

Because of this, health insurance companies were in need of unequivocal directives to help with screening between normal and pathological pregnancies and birth. The costs of hospital birth were only paid when there were medical indications, but some of the conditions for these indications were ambiguous or idiotic. Psychological indications were lacking for cases of panic when nothing medical was wrong. In 1958 the advisers of the insurance companies invited me to give a lecture about indications for hospital deliveries, and they asked me to make a record of this speech. They started to use what I'd said as a checklist for medical indications. Years later I heard that this list was called the "Kloostermanlist." Obstetricians regularly wrote me about their concerns: They would complain about an indication being omitted, or that they had a problem but could not give a referral since it was not mentioned on my list. So the list was growing and growing, and questionable indications were added to it. Besides, it was also used in another way than originally intended. In many cases, the list gave only recommendations, which guaranteed the right to a paid hospital stay, but some obstetricians were making the list obligatory: if an indication for specialist help appeared on it, the woman had to be sent to a hospital.

For these reasons, the list had to be revised. A committee was set up, which cleared the whole list, but the obstetricians did not want to accept the new list. The old one had only two categories, "yes" and "no." The new one had three: "yes," "no," and "consultation." In the third instance, midwives had final say. Some obstetricians objected to this because they considered themselves the experts, and they did not want to comply if the midwife said, "I disagree with you." I myself do not see any justification for their fears; midwives will listen to good arguments; it is in their own interest to do so.

There is always a conflict between natal and prenatal care. In Sweden, the emphasis is on natal care, which concentrated in bastions of technology, while in the Netherlands, special attention is given to prenatal care. We must admit that the Dutch organization of obstetrical care created a problem that does not exist in many other countries. There all deliveries are supposed to take place in a hospital. We try to determine during pregnancy, that is during prenatal care, which women must go to hospital and which women may choose between a home or hospital confinement. This choice became an important feature of our prenatal care.

In retrospect, it can be said that 95 percent of all pregnant women could have been confined without any assistance, but before the birth, during pregnancy, we have to be more careful and advise up to 30 percent to have their deliveries in a hospital. Dutch professors and directors of the schools for midwives have always taken that position. After good prenatal care, 70 or 80 percent of all women's pregnancies are normal: one child, good placement, the head presents, no disproportion between head and pelvis. One can say to these women: "Everything is going well." I admit that you must say to the other 20 or 30 percent: "This will become a breech birth; the head does not present. It may be better to have your baby in the hospital."

The screening between the normal and the pathological has become more and more stringent. Twenty-five years ago I expected a decrease in the number of women from the 5 percent who then had to go to a hospital during labor. That prediction did not come true. At present, almost 20 percent of the women who wanted to have their first baby at home will be sent to the hospital during labor. That increase is owing to an increased fear of risk. The number of unexpected risks decreased, however, which made the emergency cases decrease as well.

In short, the basis of our health system is that primary caretakers do the referrals: midwives are for normal deliveries, and obstetricians are for pathological births. In my opinion, that is an excellent system, but it is terribly important that there be mutually good relations between midwives and obstetricians. In the surrounding countries, obstetricians have a kind but condescending attitude towards midwives, even though they save the doctors much time. When the baby is ready to be born, midwives must call for the doctor. Afterwards, the doctor takes the credit and sends his bill. In the Netherlands, the autonomous independent midwife can rely on the sympathy and the respect of the obstetricians who work in the hospital. Some women of the 30 percent who want to have their babies at home assisted by a midwife are handed over to obstetricians just before, or even during, birth. In these instances, the woman is welcome in the hospital. Abroad, a woman will often be reproached: "How could you be so stupid as to want to have your baby at home?" Women are afraid of that kind of confrontation, and that may be a reason for some of them to stay at home too long.

Delaying the transfer to hospital causes risks that could have been avoided at an earlier moment. Such risks give obstetricians the opportunity to warn against home birth. Throughout the industrial world, home birth has thus been made to appear dangerous. That is something I reproach the obstetricians for. I see this as result of a struggle for power between a dominating masculine world and a female world. If the two camps of midwives and obstetricians face off against one another, the midwife will get the worst of it. Midwives must be careful; they must be willing and able to argue with individual obstetricians, but they should not antagonize the world of obstetricians or their professional association. I am opposed to polarization. Some people blame me for exaggerating the qualities of midwives, and that may be right, but I hope that those with less power, the women, in the long run will win.

THE FUTURE OF HOME BIRTH

In the 1950s, a delegation from the Soviet Union visiting the Netherlands asked why we still had training courses for midwives. At that time, they still had midwives, but they were very proud that soon they would be able to offer the services of obstetricians to the whole population. They thought that was the best care anyone could get. I did not agree with them. Ten years later, they still had midwives, but then home birth was forbidden. At a conference in Moscow organized by the World Health Organization, I spoke in defense of home birth. The Russians were particularly set against it, "because it was forbidden and because hospitals were better for the people." In my opinion, the reasons they were against home birth were: bad social conditions, poor housing, and above all an ideology that suited hospital births: "everyone is a child of the state, isn't he?"

And ever since, home births have decreased throughout the Western world. Sweden has been a pioneer in that respect. In the beginning of the 1960s, almost 100 percent of Swedish women had their babies in a hospital, preferably in large hospitals with more than 3,000 deliveries a year. Although technically this is defensible, from a psychological or a sociological perspective, the issue is more difficult. In the Western world, obstetricians have systematically obstructed home birth, and recently, the German obstetric association wrote a letter to all the Ministries of Health of the *Bundesländer* that contained the slogan *Schlusz mit der Hausgeburt* (stop home birth). The association set themselves up as protectors of German children, acting against the romantic ideas of some parents.

The Dutch obstetric system has become an anomaly, causing more and more amazement in surrounding countries. I defended home birth at a London congress on obstetric organization in the 1980s, which was visited by mothers-to-be, midwives, pediatricians, and obstetricians. Many obstetricians left the meeting because of lack of interest and to protest. Their actions demonstrate the emotional character of the issue. The obstetricians' criticism is becoming louder and louder. My viewpoint in favor of midwives and home birth is supported mainly by psychologists, psychiatrists, pediatricians, and sociologists. Sometimes objections to home birth in the Netherlands refer to the relatively slow decrease in perinatal mortality in the last decennia. But throughout the Western world, differences in perinatal mortality have diminished; our present-day slower decline in perinatal mortality may be explained by our earlier low perinatal mortality level.

The place of delivery is not an important factor influencing perinatal mortality. Within the Netherlands, there appears to be no correlation between regional percentages of home birth and regional perinatal mortality rates.

In 1978, I was afraid that the number of home births was diminishing beyond a critical level, but during the last fifteen years, the number of home births did not decline, while perinatal mortality continued to diminish, from 12.5 to 9.1 per thousand. Nevertheless, there is increasing pressure to give up home birth, and the impending unification of Europe may even reinforce this tendency. Besides, changing social conditions threaten the Dutch obstetric system. Some of these are high-rise buildings with twenty stories, traffic jams. These circumstances make home birth more hazardous. Another threat to the Dutch obstetric system lies in what will happen to the profession of midwife. The midwives' position may weaken with the disappearance of the old-fashioned dedication. The lifelong devotion of earlier midwives hardly exists anymore.

But I hope that home birth will endure, because there will always be some women who want to have their babies at home. They like to be self-reliant, they feel "I can work it out myself," and they prefer the intimacy of the home. My wife is one of those women, and when I asked her why she preferred to stay at home, she said that she didn't like all those strangers at her bed. All over the world, groups of this kind of woman are advocating home birth. For these people, our system may serve as an example. So, the minister of health for Ontario came here to see for himself. When he went back to Canada, he set up an experiment with lying-in clinics, good prenatal care, a good selection system, and legally recognized midwives. For implementing the Dutch system, a good infrastructure like that is necessary, with well-trained midwives who have learned to work autonomously and who are not subservient, but complementary to obstetricians.

We can only maintain our obstetric system if the international community of obstetricians becomes more tolerant towards our way of working, and women with a normal pregnancy dare to have their babies at home, while those who are at risk go to a hospital. There is some risk that the wrong people will stay at home, people who will take unacceptable risks. I want to warn against romanticism, but if we succeed in lighting the fire for home birth, our system will survive.

12

Going Dutch: Lessons for Americans

Barbara Katz Rothman

For the gardener, the real Netherlands, the heart and soul of the Netherlands, is to be found in the Keukenhof garden, a botanical garden of bulbs. There, on a spring day, standing on the walk-around of the windmill at the edge of the Keukenhof, overlooking the acres of red, gold, purple, and white bulb fields, one could be nowhere else in the world but in the Netherlands.

For the art lover, the essence of this land is to be found in one of the many, many museums. For some, it would be at the Rijksmuseum in Amsterdam, facing the classic Rembrandt *Nightwatch*. For others, it would be in one of the smaller tucked-away museums, a bicycle ride away from the train station.

But there is another place to find the heart, the soul of the Netherlands. It is up a very steep staircase. Duck under the hanging laundry crisscrossing above you—the dampness of the Lowlands is probably good for tulips, but does the laundry ever dry in this country? At the top of the stairs turn right and down the hall. Follow the sounds: voices murmuring, an occasional groan, and occasional soft laughter. Stand there quietly, for here is where the Netherlands really lives, where it is born. The midwife's light voice, the husband's voice softened, the grandmother perhaps there, the tension showing strongest in her voice. You do not have to speak the language to hear what is happening. The voices increase in their intensity, the mother's breathing harshens, she cries out, and then there is the sound of the newborn's greeting wail.

For those concerned with childbirth, and especially for those of us dedicated to alternatives in childbirth, the Netherlands has always stood as the point of reference: the goal, the proof, the argument. Mecca for Midwives. That it works there proves that it can work. It? The elusive "good birth."

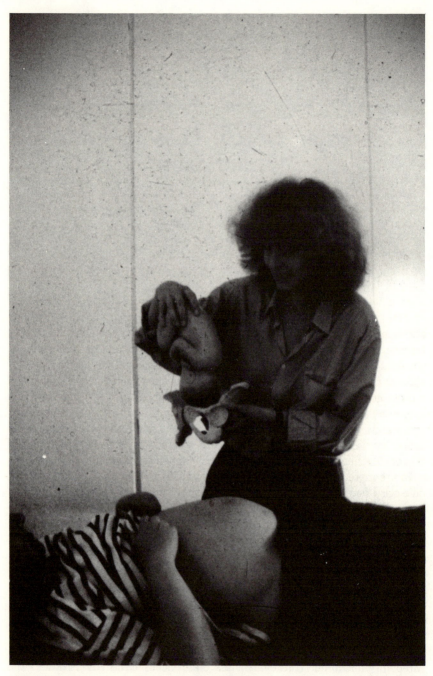

Midwife Astrid Limburg using a doll to explain the position of the fetus during birth. Used by permission of Astrid Limburg.

In reviewing childbirth practices in the Netherlands, I want to be your guide in a world that is so fundamentally different that all of our taken-for-granted assumptions may be challenged. That birth is different in different places is itself the first challenge. The United States' dependence on the hospital as a place of birth encourages us to think of birth as apart from daily life. If one thinks of birth in a narrow medical sense, one focuses on fetal parts, maternal abdomens and pelvises, and there is a certain baby-out-of-vagina sameness in it all. A pelvic arch is a pelvic arch, a fontenel a fontenel the world over, but it is women who give birth, women's vaginas, pelvises, and abdomens being probed and measured and palpated and swabbed. These women are people, with political, social, occupational, and family position in the society.

Teeth, tongue, jaw, intestines are all pretty much the same the world over, but the meaning of a meal could not be more different as we move from a famine in Ethiopia to a "food court" in a suburban mall, from a Passover seder to a fast-food lunch, from a Chinese banquet to a steakhouse in Chicago. So it is with childbirth: the social and cultural variation overwhelms the physical sameness.

Even within the United States, birth is hardly homogeneous. If the person-from-Mars, that outside observer, came to see births here, what she would probably notice as the biggest difference among birthing women is the class difference. Birth for poor women in the United States is indeed very different from birth for wealthy women. There are of course the dramatic differences in the amenities: a private room in a private hospital looks nothing like a four-bed room in an inner-city public hospital, if indeed one is lucky enough to get that four-bed room and not be left on a stretcher in the hall. But peeling paint versus rotating art works, a shortage of blankets versus flowered sheets, dried out chicken and instant mashed potatoes versus lobster and champagne postpartum dinners—these are just a small part of the difference. Poor women are more likely to be birthing without support from family or friends; middle-class women are more likely (thanks to the successes of the childbirth reform movement) to have their husband or other partner with them. Poor women have less control over their physical privacy for the duration of the labor; poor and middle-class women alike lose much control over their physical privacy and space during the birth or "delivery." Privacy, or its lack, remains an issue for poor women in the period of hospitalization following birth. Middle-class women are more likely to be able to keep their babies with them for longer periods and keep interventions to a minimum. Most profoundly, middle-class women are more likely to have a living, healthy baby, while poor women and women of color stand a much higher chance in the United States of having a sick, damaged, dying, or dead baby.

Although undoubtedly there are class differences in the Netherlands as well, the observer here is struck by how small those differences seem. Alongside private insurance, there is a national insurance program that gives everyone access to coverage. The private/public care distinction does not exist in the same way as it does in the United States, and it is not only in medical care that class differences are muted: other social support services exist in ways that people here are not used to. Moroccan immigrant families, who are among the newest and poorest of the Dutch people, live in decent apartments, pleasantly arranged and not so strikingly different to the uninformed American eye than the homes of more well-to-do, better-educated, native-born Dutch people. Compare that with the enormous housing problems, up to and including homelessness, faced by both native-born poor and immigrant poor women in the United States. Dutch women do not have to face homes without heat in the winter, without safety, with ceilings falling on them, with lead paint peeling off the woodwork, with roaches, and with rats running wild in the halls.

Thus, at the very broadest level, the Dutch have a very different approach to protecting and providing for their citizenry than we do in the United States. This protection extends to women in their role as mothers and in their role as workers. The women of the Netherlands are, as are most women in the world, given long periods of paid maternity leave before (six weeks) as well as after childbirth (ten weeks). That is a world apart from the situation most women here face, where there is no paid leave at all, or at best, a six weeks' total of "disability" and "sick" leave. Colleagues in the Netherlands had a difficult time understanding that even as a tenured professor in a major university, I was entitled to no paid leave with the birth or adoption of a child. Had I been able to afford it, I could have taken a semester off, however, and then returned to my job. That is better than most women's options in the United States. Far from a guarantee of an ongoing salary, most women here have no guarantee that their job will be waiting for them when they need to return to work: *unpaid maternity leave is still a matter of debate in the United States.*

One could of course provide this kind of basic decency, the "safety net," welfare programs, whatever they are called: housing, income protection, job protection, medical care, and still have highly medicalized, hospital-based, obstetrician-controlled births. That is the route that most of the rest of the developed world has taken. The United States is exceptional in its absence of health-care coverage, lack of paid maternity leave, and depth of poverty of some of its people.

What the Netherlands provides that is unique is an empowered midwifery. There the midwife is an independent professional, *not* practicing under the auspices, watchful eye, or control of obstetricians. Dutch midwives, as pointed out repeatedly in this book, are independent professionals who call upon obstetrician specialists for referral and consultations as needed, and most important, it is the *midwife* who makes the decision about what is needed.

Let us think about what that comes to mean in concrete settings. Dutch midwives have what in the United States is called "admitting privileges." They can admit a woman to the hospital and be her primary provider. That is rarely the case here: although nurse-midwives are often the employees of hospitals, their practices are curtailed by hospital policy. Nonnurse, lay, or empirical midwives most often may only refer a woman to an obstetrician, ask for a consultation, and then either turn the case over to the obstetrician or thank that specialist for his/her help and continue being the provider of care for the birthing woman.

For those readers who have had experience with the home birth movement in the United States, think about what it means: if a transfer is necessary, a home birth here can be a disaster, emotionally if not physically. The midwife may not even be able to accompany the woman inside the hospital door, but has to abandon her at the entrance. For my second home birth, we joked that if there was a complication, I was going to stick a hat on my midwife, claim she was my husband, and hang on tight. *Abandon* is really the apt word here: the hospital staff is often punitive, angry, and hostile towards the woman who has attempted a home birth. Horror stories abound. I think of the woman who went to have a small tear repaired after the birth, and had a nurse screaming at her that she was irresponsible, that her baby (at home in loving arms) was probably dead. Where does such anger come from? Could it be feelings of rejection because the woman dared to think that she did not need medical services? A spurned lover could be no more vicious.

The threat of a transfer, of being "screened out," hangs over every attempt at anything other than a standard medical birth in the United States. Women here, and their midwives, look to such criteria not as a simple safety issue, but, rightly, as a political barrier. Blood levels need to stay within certain parameters—maybe that is to ensure a healthy baby, but it also helps to stay within the home birth or birth center care. Weeks of gestation are carefully monitored—going late might indicate a problem with the baby, but it probably does not. What it does mean is not being able to have your baby at home. Techniques for gently bringing on labor are circulated among home birthers, the overarching concern not being for the baby (who, after all, has been in there for nine months, and if all signs are good, will not mind another two days), but to ensure the mother can have her baby at home, where she wants to have it. A woman attempting home birth in the United States is always aware that that is what she is doing: *attempting*. The spectre of failure dominates every discussion.

Transfer to medical care from midwifery care can work well in the United States. Especially when a woman is using a hospital-based nurse-midwifery program is this true, but some would argue that that care was in a sense medically based to begin with. Even for women using nonmedical, out-of-hospital care, however, a transfer during pregnancy can go smoothly, but a transfer in labor from a home birth to a hospital birth is a leap across the world in the United States. This is not the case in the Netherlands.

It sometimes seems that every American seriously involved in the home birth movement has, if lucky and blessed, an eventual opportunity to go to the Netherlands and see a home birth. It is a kind of rite of passage for the childbirth afficionado. My first Dutch home birth experience began just as it should, up to and including the laundry in the stairwell, the barking dog, the young woman with a tattooed arm, her boyfriend looking nervous, and her pacing mother. "Now," the midwife said, "now, you can see how it is really done, how Dutch women know how to give birth, how we're not infected with your American fear." It ended several hours later at the hospital with the obstetrician coming in, conferring with the midwife, briefly examining the woman, and agreeing to do a Caesarean section, or a "Caesar," as the Dutch say.

In between, there are flashes in my mind of what happened. The labor was not progressing, and the midwife became concerned. Perhaps bladder pressure was a problem. She tried a catheter, change of position, more time, more changes. Then the decision to move to the hospital: helping the woman slip some clothes on, all of us helping her maneuver down those stairs, placing her in the car next to her boyfriend, waving goodbye to the worried grandmother-to-be, jumping in the car with the midwife, and the two cars going off to the hospital. I remember holding the hospital door open for the midwife, carrying one of her bags while she carried another, with a birth stool tucked under her arm. There was a friendly welcome at the entrance, and a warmer welcome from the nurse on duty. A brief exchange of information, and the nurse set things up the way the midwife liked them—an experienced team comfortably working together. More time, more changes of position. I found myself alone by the side of the laboring woman, who was stretched out on a padded table, crying in a Dutch that even I could understand, "I want to go to sleep; let me sleep." Reassuring her (in English—who knows what a laboring woman understands of a language she studied in high school?), but aiming for the right tone of compassion and assurance, I said the midwife would be right back, "She's coming; she'll be right here." Then finally, the consultation, the goodbyes, and the midwife assuring the woman and the boyfriend that things were now okay. She said she would see them tomorrow, and off we went.

How we argued in the car going back! "How could you just *leave* her there," I demanded. "What would you have me do?" the midwife countered, the voice of reason and patience, while steering the car through the early morning empty streets. "She needed surgery and I am not a surgeon. I will see her tomorrow, answer her questions, talk to her, help her."

How truly, truly different this situation was. I knew it intellectually, but it was not until I saw it in action that I understood it and what it meant. That midwife was able to bring the woman into the hospital and keep on doing what she had been doing. Had it worked—had the woman then been able to push the baby out—the difference between a home and a hospital birth would have been largely a matter of geography. It would only have been a transfer of *place*. Although I would not have wanted to walk down that flight of stairs in labor, for the woman the descent was difficult, not traumatic. We did not transfer authority lines, worlds, value systems.

When the transfer of authority was made, from midwife care to surgical obstetric care, it was made because the woman and the midwife decided on it. Think how much that frees the midwife to transfer the woman to a hospital when she has concerns and thinks she might want surgical assistance. At every point, think how much freer the midwife is to ask for an obstetrical consult when she knows that she will not be instantly discarded, the woman automatically railroaded into a kind of birth she did not want.

I came to realize on that drive back to her home and office that the issue was trust. The midwife was transferring the woman to a trustworthy place. She had participated in the decision, had in fact made the decision, that surgery was needed, and now was trusting surgeons and their assistants to do their job. She trusted them to treat the woman decently, with kindness as well as technical competence. It was not a hostile world.

By three in the morning, arguments and tension behind us, we laughed. Oh, how we laughed! So much for my Dutch home birth experience. For this I went to the Netherlands from the United States, Caesarean section capital of the world. I traveled there for a chance to observe a woman have a Caesarean, but in fact it was infinitely more informative in its way than a "good birth" would have been, or even the good Dutch home births I later got to see. I had had two good births myself at home and seen a few more in the United States. A good American home birth is not very different from a good Dutch one. The main change is that here everyone is aware of how unusual it is, and there is a sense of pride in doing it, of having won the battle and made it through. Perhaps it can be said of births, as Leo Tolstoy said of families, the happy ones are all the same; it is the unhappy ones that are interesting.

I cannot overlook completely, however, the difference between Dutch births and births here, even when they are both home births. While having a home birth here usually feels like an accomplishment that has been wrested from an unwilling system, a Dutch home birth is part of a long and valued tradition. This means that the parameters for understanding and evaluating the situation are different as well: if one does not achieve a home birth by grit, courage, and determination, then not having a home birth is in no way a failure of these qualities. Think of same-day surgery centers: once they became widely available and encouraged by insurance providers as a cheaper form of care, outpatient cataract surgery, for example, became distinctly less traumatic for the patient. In this type of surgery, however, if there is a complication afterwards, having to go to the hospital says nothing about the kind of person you are. It does not make you a failure. If you *choose* in-patient care for cataract surgery—as a Dutch woman might choose a hospital birth—you are fully aware that it is a choice you made and not inherent in the nature of the procedure.

On a more homey, familiar level, the Dutch did not have to invent rituals and traditions for themselves for home births. We Americans did. In the Netherlands, I saw special crocheted covers for hot water bottles to place around the welcoming bassinet. Our home births in the 1970s had such a makeshift feel, as we had to figure out what equipment was useful and what unnecessarily mystifying. We also had to invent our family rituals of welcome, of celebration. For some, it was adapting the toast, opening a bottle of champagne, the ritual of weddings, launchings, New Years, beginnings. For others it was the birthday cake, creating the ritual of the very first birthday. The Dutch have some lovely little crackers with sprinkles as a traditional birth treat. It is special for birth; a genuinely traditional ritual.

Finally, to conclude my description of Dutch birth in contrast to birth in the United States, there are the maternity home-care assistants. Whether the birth takes place in the home or a hospital, in the first, often hectic days afterwards, the family is given a maternity assistant who works in the home. She comes for the eight days following the birth. For a home birth, she is expected to arrive in time to help the midwife at the birth and is then someone who has shared the birth with the family. The maternity aide can provide practical services—answering the phone, getting young children off to school in the morning, preparing meals—that permit the mother and father to sleep, rest, and take care of the baby. This is not the "baby nurse" that readers here may be familiar with—the classic figure in starched white who guards the crib and who often forms a barricade between the mother and the rest of the family on the one hand, and her infant charge on the other.

On my first postpartum visit in the Netherlands, the door was answered by someone I took to be the baby's aunt. She was washing up from lunch and about to pick up the older child at a friend's house. She told us the mother, father, and baby were sleeping upstairs. Only later did I learn that she was the maternity aide—that this was not help one buys if rich or borrows from friends and family if not, but the birthright of all Dutch families.

The maternity care assistant not only provides household help, but the special educational services a first-time mother and father especially need—and she provides them in the optimal setting: the home in which the infant is being raised. It is one thing to learn to bathe a plastic doll in a special parent education class and a very different thing to have an experienced person with you as you bathe your own baby in your own sink for the first few times. Similarly, breast-feeding assistance in the home and family setting is far more useful than a class or counseling session, let alone the videotapes now offered by some hospitals here.

It is not just a matter of learning more or getting richer information. The messages provided by a maternity assistant in one's own home are different from those given in a class or by a counselor, however well-intentioned they may be. Offering a videotape on breast-feeding assumes that this is something one needs to learn, and by implication, it is possible not to learn how to do it: to fail. Thus, here the familiar language of "achieving breast-feeding success" includes within it the inherent notion of failure. The maternity assistant, in contrast, is there if one needs the help, but since she can also make lunch or wash the diapers, her presence does not imply the mother's incompetence.

This, then, is how birth in the Netherlands differs from birth in the United States: there is a universal access to essential services, and the belief that birth is normal pervades the system. The professional autonomy of the midwife is, one can argue, both the cause and the effect of that belief. The belief in the normality and fundamental healthiness of birth and the empowerment of the midwife not only permits birth to be healthy, but also allows intervention (from Caesarean section to shampooing the soft spot) to be used in a trusted setting. The Dutch believe that a woman will be able to give birth to her baby and to take care of it. The support and help she needs are in keeping with the rest of her life going smoothly while she attends to this most important activity. Someone else can wash her dishes, and although someone else may substitute for her at work, her own salary will continue. The Dutch woman can trust the system because the Dutch system trusts the woman.

What of the future for home birth? There are two futures at question, that of the Netherlands and that of the United States. The American or anyone else committed to home birth and independent midwifery wants to know if we can use the Netherlands as our model, adopt its policies, and transfer its systems. To the extent that enormous, potentially revolutionary social, economic, and ideological changes are possible, the answer is "yes." The key is the midwife. Midwives throughout the United States, many through the Midwives Alliance of North America, are organizing for the political power their Dutch sisters have. Their successes lie in the particularities of their states: for example, in states with large populations of poor women, midwives tend to have more success. Border midwives in Texas have astonishing degrees of autonomy compared to midwives in wealthier communities. Formerly, when midwives were the professionals most women in labor called upon, obstetricians and medical doctors had to compete with them to obtain "clinical material." Now that clinical material is not a premium, obstetricians are ready to turn those women over to the care of midwives.

Will there some day be some kind of universal health insurance system in the United States? Maybe, but universal access does not necessarily mean access to midwifery care. Some fear that a national health insurance program would lock out the midwife even further. American childbirth activists need to work in these two separate areas to ensure quality care for birthing women: access to services and the support of an independent profession of midwifery. Both are uphill battles.

The other question, in its own way even more intriguing, has to do with the future of midwifery and home birth in the Netherlands: how long can they continue to hold the line? If we lose there, what hope have we here? The challenges to midwifery and home birth in the Netherlands are clearly presented in this book, and they are concerns for childbirth activists everywhere. As I see it, the concerns lie in surprisingly disparate areas. One is the ability of Dutch obstetricians not to succumb to increasing international pressure with the unification of Europe. They will need all the support they can get to resist this pressure.

The other changes are newer areas of concern: the future of feminism and what it will mean for midwifery, and the challenge presented by the international marketing of reproductive technologies. The feminists we will always have with us. We are here, there, and everywhere. What changes is the kind of feminism that flowers in different times and places, for feminism does not speak with a single voice. At the risk of oversimplification, one can see a continued swing between a more "liberal" and a more "radical" feminism.

Radical feminism has been women-centered, valuing women's culture, women's differences, women's uniqueness. Radical feminists have worked to support the community and world of women. Midwifery is in this sense feminist praxis. The very word "midwife" means "with the woman"; it is more of an ideological and political stance than a physical location.

The liberal feminist approach has been both narrower and broader, focusing on issues of discrimination. Liberal feminism works best to defend women's rights to be like men, to enter into men's worlds and work at men's jobs for men's pay, to have the rights and privileges of men. In opening the doors of men's worlds to women, liberal feminists run the risk of emptying out the worlds of women. When women have equal access to the medical schools, will they want to be lower-paid midwives? Also, midwives in the Netherlands, for all their professional autonomy, do not stand on equal social footing with physicians. The pay differences are frankly ludicrous, explainable only by sex discrimination.

Will ongoing feminist struggle in the Netherlands work to improve the salaries of midwives, or will it open up alternatives so that women move away from midwifery? The problem is most clearly seen with maternity home-care assistants. Will women continue to go into a job that lacks prestige, authority, and a good salary? In the United States, new opportunities for women had the unintended consequence of "emptying out" certain women's fields, as women found they could make more money and work better hours if they moved out of nursing and on to the maintenance staff; they could do better for themselves painting walls than caring for patients.

Dutch midwives do indeed need to organize to protect their own interests. As women they have often been reluctant to speak for their own needs, accepting ongoing sacrifices as part of their lot. Midwives and maternity home-care assistants need to develop a new assertiveness, not moving to more prestigious and better-paying fields, but demanding these benefits for themselves. That is the radical feminist approach: not equal number of men entering midwifery, not women leaving midwifery for obstetrics, but a consolidation of women's power in women's fields.

The second challenge, as Tjeerd Tymstra shows, is for me the more worrying and more profound: The technologies of reproduction, particularly the technologies of prenatal diagnosis, are being introduced to the Netherlands. They are arriving in a marketing context. The Dutch, a relatively healthy, relatively wealthy, and relatively well-organized people for medical care, are a great untapped market for the manufacturers of prenatal diagnostic kits, drugs, and services. What will be the impact of the introduction of this technology on the Dutch ideology and practice of birth, midwifery, and motherhood? It is, to use a military analogy that seems unfortunately apt, an attack from the flank. Dutch midwives have focused on birth, on protecting the normalcy of birth itself, highlighted in home birth. The ongoing threats to home birth are familiar, with the responses well organized and well thought out.

Prenatal diagnosis brings something new: the medicalization of *pregnancy*. From the points of view of the midwives, it is their clients who are being screened when mass programs of AFP screening, ultrasound, amniocentesis, and the like become the norm. It is specifically low-risk women, young women, healthy women, who are the targets of mass screening. The testing occurs in medical settings and involves the use of ultrasound to date the pregnancy "scientifically." For American women, pregnancy has been so profoundly medicalized for so long that the introduction of yet another test may not be immediately perceived as significant. For Dutch women, many of whom go through their entire reproductive lifetimes of pregnancies and births without ever seeing an obstetrician and without ever making a hospital visit, this is a dramatic change. One question is what the medicalization of pregnancy will mean for the management of birth. One midwife shared the story of a woman she had seen through two home births. In the third pregnancy, the woman, now over the age of thirty-six, had prenatal diagnosis. An unusually shaped uterus was discovered, the woman was reclassified as "high risk," and despite two "uneventful home births" (as the physicians call it), she was hospitalized for the third.

As Tymstra shows, the problem is far greater than the more you test, the more you find. It is the beginning of a shift in thinking. The Dutch think birth is healthy. At best, Americans think most births are low risk. To call something "low risk" is to focus on the risk, and this focus moves to the kind of binary thinking Tymstra describes (if there is a risk, either it will or it will not happen; subjectively it is 50:50). To focus on risk is to enter the world of responsibility. With "anticipated decision regret" comes the imperative character of the technology.

Once pregnancy is analyzed in terms of risks and potential regrets, once the fetus has been reified on the sonogram screen, the flickering video image of the fetus becoming more real than its felt presence, birth itself is profoundly altered. With this may come the greatest challenge to Dutch midwifery so far.

Select Bibliography

Ackerknecht, E. H., "Anticontagionism between 1821 and 1867," *Bulletin of the History of Medicine*, 22 (1948): 562–593.
———, *A Short History of Medicine*. Baltimore, Md./London, Johns Hopkins University Press, 1968.
AIMS, *Choosing a Home Birth*, London: AIMS, 1986.
Albermann, Eva, "The place of birth," *British Journal of Obstetrics and Gynaecology*, 93 (July 1986): 657–658.
Albers, Leah L., and Vern L. Katz, "Birth setting for low-risk pregnancies. An analysis of the current literature," *Journal of Nurse-Midwifery* 36 (1991): 215–220.
Alment, E.A.J., A. Barr, M. Reid, and J.J.A. Reid, "Normal confinement: a domiciliary and hospital study," *British Medical Journal*, ii (1967): 530–535.
Anderson, Michael, *Approaches to the History of the Western Family 1500–1914*, London and Basingstoke: The Macmillan Press, 1980.
Anderson, Roni, and Deborah Greener, "A descriptive analysis of home births attended by CNMs in two nurse-midwifery services," *Journal of Nurse-Midwifery*, 36 (1990): 95–103.
Arms, Suzanne, *Immaculate Deception. A New Look at Women and Childbirth* (3rd ed.), New York: Bantam Books, 1981.
Barker-Benfield, G. J., *The Horrors of the Half-known Life: Male Attitudes Toward Woman and Sexuality in Nineteenth Century America*. New York: Harper and Row, 1976.
Barron, S. L., A. M. Thomson, and P. R. Philips, "Hospital and hospital confinement in Newcastle upon Tyne 1960-60," *British Journal of Obstetrics and Gynaecology*, 84 (1977): 401–411.
Burke, Peter, *Venice and Amsterdam*. London: Temple Smith, 1974.
Burnett, Claude A., James A. Jones, Judith Rooks, Chong Hwa Chen, Carl W. Tyler,

and C. Arden Miller, "Home delivery and neonatal mortality in North Carolina," *Journal of the American Medical Association*, 244 (1980): 2741–2745.

Butler, N. R, and D. G. Bonham (eds.), *Perinatal Mortality, The First Report of the
1958 Perinatal Mortality Survey.* Edinburgh/London: Livingstone, 1963.

Campbell, Rona, Isobel MacDonald Davies, Allison Macfarlane, and Valerie Beral,
"Home births in England and Wales, 1979: Perinatal mortality according to intended place of delivery," *British Medical Journal*, 289 (1982): 721–724.

Campbell, Rona, and Allison Macfarlane, "Place of delivery: a review," *British Journal
of Obstetrics and Gynaecology*, 93 (July 1986): 675–683.

Caplan, M., and R. J. Madeley, "Home deliveries in Nottingham 1980–81," *Public
Health*, 99 (1985): 307–313.

Carter, Jenny, and Thérèse Duriez, *With Child: Birth Through the Ages.* Edinburgh:
Mainstream Publishing, 1986.

Cochrane, A., *Effectiveness and Efficiency, Random Reflections on Health Services.*
Abingdon: Nuffield Provincial Hospitals Trust, 1972.

Cooter, R., "Anticontagionism and history's medical record," in *The Problem of Medical Knowledge*, Wright, P., and A. Treacher (eds.), Edinburgh: Edinburgh University Press, 1982.

Darlington, Thomas, "The present status of the midwife," *American Journal of Obstetrics and Gynecology*, 63 (1911): 870–876.

Davis, L. et al., *Cesarean section rates in low risk patients managed by nurse-
midwives and obstetricians*, XIII World Congress of Gynaecology and Obstetrics (FIGO), abstract no. 0136, Singapore, 1991.

Dennis, J., and I. Chalmers, "Very early neonatal seizure rate: a possible epidemiological indicator of the quality of perinatal care." *British Journal of Obstetrics
and Gynaecology*, 89, 1982, 418–426.

Department of Health and Social Security (DHSS), *Report on Confidential Enquiries
into Maternal Deaths in England and Wales 1967–69.* London: DHSS, 1972.

Devitt, Neal, "The statistical case for elimination of the midwife: fact versus prejudice, 1890–1935," *Women and Health*, 4 (1979): 81–96, 169–186.

DeVries, Raymond G., *Regulating Birth: Midwives, Medicine and the Law.* Philadelphia: Temple University Press, 1985.

Dexter, Margaret, and Wally Harbert, *The Home Help Service.* London/New York:
Tavistock Publications, 1983.

Donegan, James B., *Women and Men Midwives: Medicine, Morality, and Misogyny
in Early America.* Westport Conn.: Greenwood Press, 1978.

Donnison, Jean, *Midwives and Medical Men: A History of Inter-Professional Rivalries
and Women's Rights.* New York: Schocken, 1977.

Elias, Norbert, *Ueber den Prozess der Zivilisation.* Bern & Munich: Francke Verlag,
1969 (1938).

Eskes, T.K.A.B., H. W. Jongsma, and P.C.W. Houx, "Umbilical cord gases in home deliveries versus hospital-based deliveries," *Journal of Reproductive Medicine*, 26
(1981): 405–408.

Fleury, P. M., *Maternity Care. Mothers' Experience of Childbirth.* London: Allen and
Unwin, 1967.

Flexner, A., *Medical Education in Europe.* New York: Carnegie Foundation, Bulletin
no. 6, 1912.

Forbes, Th. R., "Midwifery and witchcraft," *Journal of the History of Medicine and Applied Sciences*, 17 (1962): 264–283.

———, "The regulation of English midwives in the sixteenth and seventeenth centuries," *Medical History*, 8 (1964): 135–244.

Gélis, Jacques, *L'arbre et le fruit: la naissance dans l'Occident moderne* (XVIe–XIXe siècle). Paris: Fayard, 1984.

Freidson, E. *Profession of Medicine. A Study of the Sociology of Applied Knowledge.* New York: Dodd, Mead, 1975.

Garcia, Jo, Beátrice Blondel, and Marie J. Saurel-Cubizolles, "The needs of childbearing families: social policies and the organization of health care," in *Effective Care in Pregnancy and Childbirth*, vol. 1, Chalmers, Ian, Murray Enkin, and Marc J. Keirse (eds.), Oxford: Oxford University Press, 1989.

Gerson, G. L., "Divided we stand: physiologists and clinicians in the American context," in *The Therapeutic Revolution*, Vogel, J., and C. E. Rosenberg (eds.), University of Pennsylvania Press, 1979, 67–91.

Golding, Jean, and N. R. Butler, "Studies of perinatal mortality: contrasts and contradictions," in *Social and Biological Effects on Perinatal Mortality*, vol. III: Perinatal Analysis. Report on an International Comparative Study Sponsored by the World Health Organization. Golding, J. (ed.), Bristol: University of Bristol Printing Unit, 1990.

Goudsblom, Johan, *Dutch Society.* New York: Random House, 1968.

Gubalke, W., *Die Hebamme in Wandel der Zeiten.* Hannover: Staude, 1964.

Having a Baby in Europe. Copenhagen: World Health Organization, 1985.

Hiddinga, Anja, "Obstetrical research in the Netherlands in the nineteenth century," *Medical History*, 31 (1987): 281–305.

Huizinga, Johan, *Herfsttij der Middeleeuwen.* Groningen: Wolters-Noordhoff, 1984 (1919).

Johnson, T., *Professions and Power.* London, Macmillan, 1972.

Jordan, Brigitte, *Birth in Four Cultures.* Montreal: Eden Press Women's Publications, 1978.

———, "Technology and the social distribution of knowledge: issues for primary health care in developing countries," in *Anthropology and Primary Health Care*, Coreil, Jeannine and J. D. Mull (eds.), Boulder: Westview Press, 1990: 98–120.

Keirse, M.J.N.C., "Interaction between primary and secondary antenatal care, with particular reference to the Netherlands," in *Effectiveness and Satisfaction in Antenatal Care*, Enkin, M., and I. Chalmers (eds.), London: Spastics International Medical Publications, Heinemann Medical Books, 1982, 222–233.

Kent, Francis W., *Household and Lineage in Renaissance Florence: The Family Life of the Capponi, Ginori, and Rucellai.* Princeton: Princeton University Press, 1977.

Kitzinger, Sheila, *Birth at Home.* Oxford: Oxford University Press, 1980.

———, "Editorial," *International Home Birth Movement Newsletter* (British Section), 1, no.1 (1990): 1–2.

Kleiverda, G., A. M. Steen, I. Andersen, P. E. Treffers, and E. Everaerd, "Place of delivery in the Netherlands: maternal motives and background variables related to preferences for home or hospital confinement," in *European Journal of Obstetrics, Gynaecology and Reproductive Biology*, 36 (1990): 1–9.

Kloosterman, G. J., "The Dutch system of home births," in *The Place of Birth*, Kitzinger, Sheila, and J. A. Davis (eds.), Oxford: Oxford University Press, 1978, 85–92.

Kobrin, Frances, "The American midwife controversy: a crisis in professionalization," *Bulletin of the History of Medicine*, 40 (1966): 158.

Laget, Mireille, *Naissance, l'accouchement avant l'age de la clinique*. Paris: Editions du Seuil, 1982.

Leavitt, Judith Walzer, *Brought to Bed: Childbearing in America, 1750–1950*. New York and Oxford: Oxford University Press, 1986.

Leavitt, Judith Walzer, and W. Walton, "Down to death's door: women's perception of childbirth in America," in *Women and Health in America*, Leavitt, J. Walzer (ed.), Madison/London, 1984, 155–166.

Lemaine, G. et al., *Perspectives on the Emergence of Scientific Disciplines*. The Hague/Paris: Mouton, 1976.

Lewis, Jane, *The Politics of Motherhood: Child and Maternal Welfare in England, 1900–1939*. London: Croom Helm, 1980.

Lievaart, M. and P. A. De Jong, "Neonatal morbidity in deliveries conducted by midwives and gynecologists: a study of the system of obstetric care prevailing in the Netherlands," *American Journal of Obstetrics and Gynecology* 152, 1985, 376–386.

MacIntyre, S., "The management of childbirth: A review of sociological research issues," *Social Science and Medicine*, 11 (1977): 477–484.

McKeown, Th., *The Modern Rise of Population*. London: Edward Arnold, 1976.

Mead, Margaret, *Sex and Temperament in Three Primitive Societies*. New York: William Morrow, 1935.

Mead, Margaret, and Niles Newton, "Cultural patterning of perinatal behavior," in *Childbearing: Its Social and Psychological Aspects*, Richardson A., and Alan F. Guttmacher (eds.), Williams & Wilkins, 1967.

Mehl, Lewis E., Gail H. Peterson, Michael Whitt, and Warren E. Hawes, "Outcomes of elective home births: A series of 1,146 cases," *Journal of Reproductive Medicine* 19 (1977): 281–290.

Mendelsohn, E., "The social construction of scientific knowledge," in *The Social Production of Scientific Knowledge*, Mendelsohn, E., and P. Weingart (eds.), Dordrecht: Reidel, 1977, 3–27.

Ministry of Health, *Enquiry into the Cost of the National Health Service* (Chairman: C. W. Guillebaud), London: HMSO, 1956.

———, *Report of the Committee on Maternity Services* (Chairman: the Earl of Cranbrook), London: HMSO, 1959.

Monagle, R. N., "Relationship of birth outcome to health care provider," *American Journal of Obstetrics and Gynecology*, 146 (1983): 870–871.

Murphy, J. F., Marjorie Dauncey, O. P. Gray, and I. Chalmers, "Planned and unplanned deliveries at home: implications of a changing ratio," *British Medical Journal*, 288 (1984): 1429–1432.

Newson, Katherine, "Direct entry method of training midwives in three countries, 1. The Netherlands," *Midwives Chronicle & Nursing Notes* (Feb. 1981): 39–43.

Oakley, Ann, *The Captured Womb: A History of the Medical Care of Pregnant Women*. Oxford: Basil Blackwell Publisher Ltd., 1984.

Olsen, Donald J., "Urbanity, modernity, and liberty: Amsterdam in the seventeenth century," in *Time and the City & Urbanity, Modernity, and Liberty*. Amsterdam: Centre for Metropolitan Research, 1988/1990: 19–41.

Pel, J., and P. E. Treffers, "The reliability of the result of the umbilical cord pH," *Journal of Perinatal Medicine*, vol. 11 (1983): 169–174.

Petersen, William, "Family subsidies in the Netherlands," *Marriage and Family Living*, XVII (1955): 260–266.

Pollock, Linda, *Forgotten Children: Parent-Child Relations from 1500–1900*. Cambridge: Cambridge University Press, 1983.

Prechtl, H.F.R., and D. J. Beintema, "The neurological examination of the full term newborn infant," in *Clinics in Developmental Medicine*, no. 12, London: Heinemann Medical Books, 1964.

Prentice, A., and T. Lind, "Fetal heart rate monitoring during labour: too frequent intervention, too little benefit? *Lancet* ii (1987): 1375–1377.

Price, Frances V., "Who helps?" in *Three, Four, and More: A Study of Triplet and Higher Order Births*, Botting, Beverley J., Allison J. Macfarlane, and Frances V. Price (eds.), London: HMSO, 1990.

Rooks, J. P. et al., "Outcomes of care in birth centers: The National Birth Center Study," *New England Journal of Medicine*, 321 (1989): 1804–1811.

Rothman, Barbara Katz, *The Tentative Pregnancy, Prenatal Diagnosis and the Future of Motherhood*. New York: Viking, 1986; Norton, 1993.

_____, *Recreating Motherhood, Ideology and Technology in a Patriarchal Society*. New York: W. W. Norton & Company, 1989.

Schama, Simon, *The Embarrassment of Riches: An Interpretation of Dutch Culture in the Golden Age*. New York: Knopf, 1987.

Scherjon, Sicco, "A comparison between the organization of obstetrics in Denmark and the Netherlands," *British Journal of Obstetrics and Gynaecology*, 93 (July 1986): 684–689.

Schneider, Dona, "Planned out-of-hospital births, New Jersey, 1978–1980," *Social Science Medicine*, 23 (1986): 1011–1015.

Schramm, Wayne F., Diane E. Barnes, and Janice M. Bakewell, "Neonatal mortality in Missouri home births, 1978–84," *American Journal of Public Health* 77 (1987): 930–935.

Shearer, J.M.L., "Five year prospective survey of risk of booking for a home birth in Essex," *British Medical Journal*, 291 (1985): 1478–1480.

Shorter, Edward, *The Making of the Modern Family*. London: Collins, 1976 (1975).

_____, *A History of Women's Bodies*. New York: Basic Books, 1982.

Simmer, H. H., "Principles and problems of medical undergraduate education in Germany during the nineteenth and early twentieth century," in *The History of Medical Education*, C. D. O'Malley (ed.), UCLA Forum of Medical Science, no. 12, Los Angeles: University of California Press, 1970, 173–200.

Smulders, Beatrijs, and Astrid Limburg, "Obstetrics and midwifery in the Netherlands," in *The Midwife Challenge*, Kitzinger, Sheila (ed.), London: Pandora Press, 1988.

Snapper, I., "Midwifery, past and present," *Bulletin of the New York Academy of Medicine,* 39 (1963): 503–532.

Stone, Lawrence, *The Family, Sex and Marriage in England 1500–1800.* Harmondsworth: Pelican, 1979 (1977).

Sullivan, Deborah A., and Rose Weitz, *Labor Pains: Modern Midwives and Home Birth.* New Haven/London: Yale University Press, 1988.

Tew, Marjorie, "Intended place of delivery and perinatal outcome (letter)," *British Medical Journal,* 91 (1978): 1139–1140.

———, "Do obstetric intranatal interventions make birth safer?" *British Journal of Obstetrics and Gynaecology,* 93 (1980): 659–674.

———, *Safer Childbirth? A Critical History of Maternity Care.* London: Chapman and Hall, 1990.

Tew, Marjorie, and S.M.J. Damstra-Wijmenga, "Safest birth attendants: recent Dutch evidence," *Midwifery* 7 (1991): 55–63.

Torres, A., and Reich, M. R., "The shift from home to institutional childbirth: A comparative study of the United Kingdom and the Netherlands," *International Journal of Health Services,* 19 (1989): 405–414.

Towler, Jean, and Joan Bramall, *Midwives in History and Society.* London: Croom Helm, 1986.

Treffers, P. E., and R. Laan, "Regional perinatal mortality and regional hospitalization at delivery in the Netherlands," *British Journal of Obstetrics and Gynaecology,* 93 (July 1986): 690–693.

Treffers, P. E., D. van Alten, and M. Pel, "Condemnation of obstetric care in the Netherlands," *American Journal of Obstetrics and Gynaecology* 146, 1983, 871–872.

Treffers, P. E. et al., "Home births and minimal medical interventions," *Journal of the American Medical Association,* 264, 1990, 2203–2208.

Tymstra, Tj., C. Bajema, J. R. Beekhuis, and A. Mantingh, "Women's opinions on the offer and use of prenatal diagnosis," *Prenatal Diagnosis* 11 (1991): 893–898.

———, "The imperative character of medical technology and the meaning of anticipated decision regret," *International Journal of Technology Assessment in Health Care,* 5 (1991): 207–213.

van Alten, D., M. Eskes, and P. E. Treffers, "Midwifery in the Netherlands; the Wormerveer study: selection, mode of delivery, perinatal mortality and infant morbidity," *British Journal of Obstetrics and Gynaecology,* 96, 1989, 656–662.

van Daalen, Rineke, "The state of infant health care in Amsterdam: Medicalization and the role of the state," *Netherlands Journal of Sociology,* 21 (2) (October 1985): 126–140.

Van Lieburg, M. J., and Hilary Marland, "Midwife regulation, education, and the practice in the Netherlands during the nineteenth century," *Medical History,* 33 (1989 A): 296–317.

van Teijlingen, Edwin R., "The profession of maternity home care assistant and its significance for the Dutch midwifery profession," *International Journal of Nursing Studies,* 27, no. 4 (1990): 355–366.

Wald, N. J., H. S. Cuckle, J. W. Densem et al., "Maternal serum screening for Down's syndrome in early pregnancy," *British Medical Journal,* 297 (1988): 883–887.

Watkin, B., *Documents on Health and Social Services, 1834 to the Present Day.* London: Methuen & Co. Ltd., 1975.

Wertz, Dorothy, and Richard Wertz, *Lying In: A History of Childbirth in America.* New York: The Free Press, 1977.

Wrightson, Keith, *English Society 1580–1680.* New Brunswick, N.J.: Rutgers University Press, 1982.

Zborowski, Mark, "Cultural components in responses to pain," *Journal of Social Issues,* 8 (4) (1952): 16–30.

_____, *People in Pain.* San Francisco: Jossey-Bass, 1969.

Index

About the Editor and Contributors

EVA ABRAHAM-VAN DER MARK is an anthropologist, currently employed at the Anthropological-Sociological Institute of the University of Amsterdam. She has published extensively in the areas of families, the role of women, and ethnicity in the Caribbean, as well as in the areas of medical anthropology and urban anthropology in the Netherlands. Her most recent publications include: "Vroedvrouwen in Nederland, een 'low tech' medische beroepsgroep" ("Midwives in the Netherlands, a Low Tech Medical Profession"), in *De macht der dingen, medische technologie in cultureel perspectief* (*The Power of Medical Technology in Cultural Perspective*), edited by Sjaak van der Geest, Paul ten Have, Gerhard Nijhof, and Piet Verbeek (1993); "Caught in the Shift: The Impact of Industrialization on Female-Headed Households in Curaçao, Netherlands Antilles," in *Where Did All the Men Go? Female-Headed/Female Supported Households in Cross-Cultural Perspective*, edited by Joan Mencher and Anne Okongwu (1993); and "Marriage and Concubinage, Women in the Sephardic Merchant Elite of Curaçao," in *Women and Change in the Caribbean*, edited by Janet Momsen (1993).

SIMONE E. BUITENDIJK is a medical doctor and director of the Foundation for Perinatal Epidemiology in the Netherlands. Among her recent publications are: "Diethylstilbestrol and the next generation: a challenge to the evidence?" in *Side Effects of Drugs Annual* (1988); "Medication Use in Early Pregnancy: Prevalence of Use and Relationship to Maternal Characteristics" (with M. B. Bracken), in *American Journal of Obstetrics and Gynecology* (1991); "Current Treatments to Prevent Miscarriages and Premature Labour in DES-daughters and Other Women," in *European Journal of Public Health* (1991); and "Non-differential Underestimation May Cause Threshold Effect of Exposure to Appear as a Dose-Response Relationship" (with P. Verkerk), in *Journal of Clinical Epidemiology* (1992).

RINEKE VAN DAALEN currently works in the department of sociology at the University of Amsterdam. She is engaged in research into the welfare state, especially the relationship between intimate, private relations and developments in the public domain of the welfare state. She has written several articles on pregnancy, birth, and the care of young children in the Netherlands, including "Van moederschapsbescherming tot ouderschapsverlof," in *Gezondheid en Samenleving* (1982); "The Start of Infant Health Care in Amsterdam: Medicalization and the Role of the State," in *The Netherlands' Journal of Sociology* (1985); "Dutch Midwifery and Childbirth: A Profile," in *Midwives Information and Resource Service (MIDIRS)* (1987); "Dutch Obstetric Care: Home or Hospital, Midwife or Gynaecologist," in *Health Promotion* (1988); and "De groei van de ziekenhuisbevalling. Nederland en het buitenland," in *Amsterdams Sociologisch Tijdschrift* (1988).

REINIE VAN GOOR is a television producer for Immigrant Television and has published *Vrouwen vertellen over de geboorte van hun kind* (*Women Talk about the Birth of Their Child*), 1990.

ANJA HIDDINGA teaches in the Department of Science Dynamics at the University of Amsterdam. She works in the areas of science and technology studies, history of medicine, and women's studies. Among her recent publications are: "X-ray Technology in Obstetrics: Measuring Pelves at the Yale School of Medicine," in *Medical Innovations in Historical Perspective*, edited by J. V. Pickstone (1992), and (with S. Blume) "Technology, Science, and Obstetric Practice: The Origins and Transformation of Cephalo-Pelvimetry," in *Science, Technology, and Human Values* (1992).

BRIGITTE JORDAN is Senior Research Scientist at the Institute for Research on Learning in Palo Alto, California, as well as a member of the Research Staff in the Work Practice and Technology Area of the Systems and Practice Laboratory at Xerox Palo Alto Research Center. Among her most recent works are: *Birth in Four Cultures: A Crosscultural Investigation of Childbirth in Yucatan, Holland, Sweden, and the United States* (1992); "Technology and the Social Distribution of Knowledge: Issues for Primary Health Care in Developing Countries," in *Anthropology and Primary Health Care*, edited by Jeanine Corell and Dennis Mull (1990); "Cosomopolitical Obstetrics: Some Insights from the Training of Traditional Midwives," in *Social Science and Medicine*; and "Childbirth Crossculturally," in *The Women's Encyclopedia*, edited by Helen Tierney (1989, Greenwood Press).

BARBARA KATZ ROTHMAN is Professor of Sociology at the City University of New York, Baruch College and the Graduate Center. Her most recent publications include: *Recreating Motherhood* (1989); *The Tentative Pregnancy* (1993); and *In Labor* (1991).

L. H. LUMEY is currently Senior Epidemiologist in the Department of Clinical Epidemiology and Biostatistics and Staff Research Scientist in the Departments of Obstetrics and Neonatology in the Academic Medical Center in Amsterdam, the Netherlands. One of his recent publications is: "Decreased Birthweight in Infants after Maternal In-Utero Exposure to the Dutch Famine of 1942-1944," in *Paediatric and Prenatal Epidemiology*, 1992.

HILARY MARLAND is a Research Officer at the Medical History Institute of the Erasmus University in Rotterdam, the Netherlands. Her research interests include the history of preventive medicine in the Netherlands, women medical practitioners, and the history of Dutch midwives, 1700–1945. Among her publications are: *Medicine and Society in Wakefield and Huddersfield, 1780–1870* (1987); *"Mother and Child Were Saved," The Memoirs of the Frisian Midwife Catharina Schrader (1693–1740)*—co-author. She has edited *The Art of Midwifery, Early Modern Midwives in Europe* (1993); and (with Valerie Fildes) *Women and Children First, International Maternal and Infant Welfare, 1870–1945* (1992).

EDWIN R. VAN TEIJLINGEN is Research Associate in the Department of General Practice at the University of Edinburgh, Scotland. His recent publications include: "The Organisation of Maternity Care in the Netherlands," in *The Association for Community-based Maternity Care Newsletter* (1992); "Going Dutch—The Profession of Maternity Home Care Assistant," in *Maternity Action* (1991); "Maternity Care in Rural Areas in the Netherlands," in *Maternity Action* (1990); "The Profession of Maternity Home Care Assistant and Its Significance for the Dutch Midwifery Profession," in *International Journal of Nursing Studies* (1990); and "The Profession of Midwife in the Netherlands" (with P. McCaffery) in *Midwifery* (1987).

PIETER E. TREFFERS is Professor of Obstetrics and Gynecology at the University of Amsterdam in the Netherlands. Among his recent publications are: "Midwifery in the Netherlands: The Wormerveer Study: Selection, Mode of Delivery, Perinatal Mortality, and Infant Morbidity" (with D. van Alten and M. Eskes), in *British Journal of Obstetrics and Gynecology* (1989); and "Home Births and Minimal Medical Interventions" (with M. Eskes, G. Kleiverda, and D. van Alten), in *Journal of the American Medical Association* (1990).

TJEERD TYMSTRA is a medical sociologist at the University of Groningen in the Netherlands. He studies the psychological impact of new medical technologies (reproductive technologies, screening procedures, organ donation, and transplantation), and recently conducted a survey of health professionals and consumers that focused on the "limits of medicine." His recent publications include: "Prenatal Diagnosis, Prenatal Screening, and the Rise of the Tentative Pregnancy," in *International Journal of Technology Assessment in Health Care* (1991); and (with J. W. Heyink, J. Pruim, and M.J.H. Sloof) "Experience of Bereaved Relatives Who Granted or Refused Permission for Organ Donation," in *Family Practice* (1992).